SUPER
HERBS

SUPER HERBS

The best adaptogens to reduce stress and
improve health, beauty and wellness

RACHEL LANDON
Illustrations by Lerryn Korda

piatkus

PIATKUS

First published in Great Britain in 2017 by Piatkus

1 3 5 7 9 10 8 6 4 2

Copyright © Rachel Landon 2017
Illustrations by Lerryn Korda

The moral right of the author has been asserted.

A CIP catalogue record for this book
is available from the British Library.

ISBN 978-0-349-41602-1

Typeset in Caslon by M Rules
Printed and bound in Great Britain by
Clays Ltd, St Ives plc

Papers used by Piatkus are from well-managed forests
and other responsible sources.

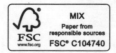

MIX
Paper from
responsible sources
FSC® C104740

Piatkus
An imprint of
Little, Brown Book Group
Carmelite House
50 Victoria Embankment
London EC4Y 0DZ

An Hachette UK Company
www.hachette.co.uk

www.improvementzone.co.uk

Disclaimer
*The information in this book is not intended to replace or conflict with the advice given
to you by your GP or other health professionals. All matters regarding your health
should be discussed with your GP. The author and publisher disclaim any liability
directly or indirectly from the use of the material in this book by any person.*

To my dear mum, Agnes Beryl, and my family: Charlie, Grace, Lou, Harps and Otis ... thank you.

Contents

Introduction

A Bit About Me

When I was a little girl my mum, who was forever practical, would point out all the different leaves and flowers in our garden and along the hedgerows that I could rub on my grazed knees and itchy insect bites. She would make a compress of distilled witch hazel, which she kept in a bottle behind the kitchen radio for all our bumps and bruises – I can still remember its astringent smell. She showed me how to crush a dock leaf and rub it on my nettle rash till my skin turned green, making me feel like I had magic at my fingertips.

I loved the connection that these precious interactions brought me and my mum, outside in nature where we'd silently pick blackberries along the railway track in the fields behind our house, and build bonfires in the autumn months, checking first for any hibernating hedgehogs. It was a complete contrast to the woman I knew most of the time. Mum's life was a tour de force: one was an older mother than most in the 1970s, a successful businesswoman, plus a single mum of four. As a young woman she had lived through the Second World War and had understood the need to be self-sufficient, and somehow, within her incredibly busy life, she still found the time to become a proficient seasonal gardener. Our home was in the North West, a half hour's drive from Manchester, and was once a farm and in between the ivy-clad barns, the disused pigsties and the rose garden, she found a plot to grow all our fruit and vegetables in long rows, surrounded by clay borders.

One of my jobs, apart from collecting eggs from Farmer Worsley two doors down, was to go out and pull up potatoes or pick green beans for our tea. This was an idyllic time for me, sitting on my own on the steps outside our back door in the evening summer sun, topping and tailing the stubbly goose-berries and shelling fresh peas from their pods with my thumb, eating more than went into the bowl. We'd spend weekend after-noons netting the raspberries to protect them from the young rooks that nested in the big oaks above. This small knowledge of nature was healing and the catalyst that started my bigger love affair with herbs.

Today I have four children of my own – from teenager to baby – all with different emotional and practical needs, and I try to support them with herbal preparations, flower remedies, homeopathy and handmade balms. My ten-year-old loves the jars of dried herbs and amber bottles of herbal tinctures, bees-wax and essential oils. He thinks it's very magical, and although we're living in London, I try to show them all wild herbs in the hedgerows every season: nettle leaves and wild garlic in early Spring, yarrow and blackberries in late Summer, and sweet chestnuts and hawthorn berries on short Winter days. I try and keep them connected to their natural environment – we just have to look a little bit harder sometimes.

My journey to becoming a herbalist started at home with my mum, our garden and my freedom in the fields behind our house. But there was a detour after my schooling finished that started in London, then moved to Paris where I was based as a fashion model in the early 1990s. I was travelling non-stop and doing the rounds of shows in Paris, London and New York, on and off planes, in and out of airports, hotels and cities, arriving in the dead of night and waking before dawn to catch the light for the photograph.

Most of the time I felt incredibly lonely and overwhelmed, and was living on adrenalin. There were no mobiles or wi-fi, so I would have to rely on public phones in the most unlikely of places to connect with loved ones. Looking back this time was a catalyst for where I am today, but at the time I was fraught with stress. I was in my early twenties and still trying to find my feet as a woman, and this stress and high state of alert started to have an effect on my whole well-being, causing hormonal imbalances, anxiety, panic attacks and digestive problems.

Everyone around me – my agents, friends, colleagues and family – thought I was lucky to be living such a life, and the guilt for not feeling the same and not being able to enjoy the moment only added to my anxiety. At the time, no one discussed anxiety or panic attacks, especially in the modelling world where vulnerability was portrayed with confidence in 1990s fashion.

Every job became a personal challenge to see how I'd cope and when I got through it I was thrilled, and then I'd crash; I was exhausted … my adrenals were shot. My agency in Paris thought I was mad for not thinking myself so fortunate to have been chosen for influential jobs and didn't understand why I might not be coping, so I decided to try and take stock and start to support myself as best I could, starting with my diet.

Paris back then was not really into 'health food' and cooking was not often an option. There were a few juice bars and a scattering of health-food shops but you really had to search for them. I found a gem of a place in Saint Germain, behind a church in a beautiful square that served the best nutritious whole food, with a different dish every day, and my weekly visits started to have a grounding effect.

I began to look again at the herbs I grew up with and started to use them to support my digestion and sleep. I decided to take some time out to study vegetarian cooking at the Cordon Vert cookery school in England. I completed the first course but back then vegetarianism was very much egg- and pastry-based, which I knew instinctively was not the way forward for me.

The opportunity to live across the Atlantic in New York City came in 1994, when I had just turned 24 and the whole revolution in health and nutrition was happening. I felt excited about the prospect of feeling strong and in control of my own well-being and I started my journey of yoga, juicing and reading book after book on nutrition and herbal medicine to find the balance of food and herbal remedies that suited my needs. I started to take courses and for the first time felt empowered and stable in the unlikely frenetic surroundings of Manhattan and the fashion world.

After four years I returned to London, resolute in the idea of studying natural medicine, specifically herbs, working with the whole person, body, mind and spirit, using herbs, nutrition and complementary natural therapies specific to an individual's needs. Hippocrates, who is looked on as the 'father of medicine', believed *health is an expression of a harmonious balance between various components of man's nature, the environment and ways of life, nature being the physician of disease.*

Today, as well as having my practice, I'm juggling our family of six and all our daily needs, sometimes trying to listen to three different conversations at once, negotiating individuals' moods, often with very little sleep, trying to get the work and home-life balance right. It really is a fine balance and something that I know we all struggle with today.

Now in my fourth decade, having lost loved ones, managing work and personal life, trying to balance hormones and negotiate the next third of my life, I realise I experience a different kind of stress to the kind I experienced in my early years. But I'm definitely more equipped to cope. I have better nutrition; I've learnt to say no (which took a while); I know what suits me and what really doesn't; and I use herbs, especially adaptogens, to help balance hormones, keep my cardiovascular system strong, nervous system supported and my whole body system vital and connected.

As a natural health-care practitioner I feel inspired to encourage people to stay healthy and prevent illness, rather than to wait until they feel overwhelmed and unwell and then start to look for help. This is why I look to this group of herbs called adaptogens. As well as balancing positive lifestyle choices, they help us to sustain optimum health in an age when it's a constant challenge.

In this book I'd like to share with you in a concise and easy way all the benefits of these incredible superherbs, which can support the whole body system in dealing with the everyday challenges of modern living.

Adaptogens: What They Are and How They Work

Most herbs are wonderful for healing specific ailments, but adaptogens are multi-dimensional. Adaptogens, or superherbs, are a group of herbs that support and rebalance the body, allowing us to adapt to stressors whether they are physical, environmental or emotional. They have been likened to a thermostat regulating our body, calming us down when we are too stressed and boosting our energy when we are depleted, but without exhausting or draining our adrenals.

Vitality is a word that best describes optimum health or feeling heathy. One of the *Oxford Dictionary*'s definitions is 'an individual's hold on life', and vitality relates to a life force and energy. Our vitality is at its strongest when we feel healthy, glowing and full of energy. Herbalists use the term 'vital force' to explain the amount of energy within the tissues and organs of the body, and when this vitality or vital force becomes depleted through stress and exhaustion you may start to feel unwell and overwhelmed.

Adaptogens are powerful supportive herbs that can help rejuvenate and support this vital force, and in doing so they can help protect the body from disease and stress.

The word 'stress' has been overused and misunderstood. Stress is a psychological reaction to a short- or long-term situation. It's the heightened response to this situation that gets the hypothalamus and pituitary glands working, that then activate the adrenal glands to secrete the stress hormones called cortisol and adrenalin. These cause the well-known 'fight or flight' feeling, with a rise in blood pressure thus increasing the heart rate. This is all good when we really need it, as in an emergency this reaction keeps us alive and then afterwards everything returns to normal. If this becomes constant though, over stressful periods in life, the repeated onslaught of cortisol has a negative impact on all your organs and weakens the immune system, which then starts to lay the foundation for disease or imbalances.

Long-term stress causes our digestive function to become weakened, our nervous systems to be overwhelmed, and a lack of dehydroepiandrosterone (thankfully shortened to DHEA), which is a hormone made by the adrenals that helps in the production of male and female sex hormones and reproductive function, but also assists in the regulation of metabolism and energy levels. It's also known as the 'youth hormone'.

Modern-day life has so many benefits, but it's also incredibly stressful. I look at my teenage daughter and wonder how she manages as she keeps up with the many social-media platforms and the constant messaging from friends who want her attention and opinion most hours of every day. If you look around you in the street, on the train or at work, the majority of people are checking their screens in the ever-expanding world of the web.

Environmentally our food chain is being compromised by processed foods and overexposure to pesticides and soil pollution from industrial agriculture. And although our life expectancies are longer, we have seen the most dramatic increase in chronic diseases such as diabetes, cancer, obesity, dementia and depression. These illnesses are often a result of our environment and our lifestyle choices, and it's up to us to make positive changes.

I see so many patients who say they feel exhausted on a daily basis, even on waking in the morning. They carry this feeling of fatigue throughout the day. An aching body, anxiety, depression, poor digestion, poor sleep, constant colds that are hard to shake, a loss of libido and hormonal imbalances, a short temper and forgetfulness are just some of the symptoms due to exhaustion. Most of us try to use caffeine to prop ourselves up, which offers a quick spike of energy then a swift crash, which further exhausts the adrenals and only exacerbates the symptoms of feeling overwhelmed – often creating a cycle of needing more caffeine to pick you up again.

Adaptogens work in supporting the adrenals and the whole endocrine system. They help to relax and rebalance the body, resisting stress by adapting the body's response to it and increasing the body's overall vitality.

From the foods and drinks we ingest, the air we breathe and the synthetic chemicals in our beauty products, make-up and perfumes to the cleaning products and room deodorisers we use – today more than ever we're exposed to a myriad toxic chemicals that our bodies have to process, metabolise and eliminate. Together with the added intensity of modern life and the demands it makes on us with work, technology and the information overload it brings, it's not a shock to learn that chronic illnesses such as heart disease, allergies and depression are on the increase and that chronic fatigue is one of the main reasons a patient visits their GP. Modern medicine unfortunately often treats the symptoms of an illness without looking at the cause or the individual and their unique needs, whereas I find medicinal herbs support and nourish the whole person.

Adaptogen herbs work with the therapeutic actions of the entire plant on the whole body system, offering a gentle alternative to synthetic drugs, which often have a direct action on just one particular system or tissue. These herbs help to regenerate the tissues and fluids of the body during stress or illness, stimulating the body's own defensive system into action rather than just working on the symptoms and not the cause.

I believe that in order to be truly healthy there needs to be a positive balance between our physical, mental and spiritual health, as well as our interrelations with the environment we surround ourselves in. We are not just what we eat or what we take into our body, but also what we think, what we do, what we say, the relationships we have and the environment we choose to have around us. These all have a direct effect upon our overall well-being.

We have to be able to ask ourselves what's not agreeing with us or having a positive effect on our lives, and be able to recognise when there's a need to take a positive step in bringing a change. If no changes can be made due to circumstances then we must learn how best to adapt and manage a more positive way of thinking and attitude.

As the inspiring novelist and activist Maya Angelou said: '*If you don't like something change it. If you can't change it, change your attitude.*'

All you need to do is to listen to your body to find what is working for you and what's not, and to put in a little work every day in order to make beneficial differences to your health.

- Eat consciously with seasonally nutritious foods that are as close to nature as possible, steering away from processed, salty and sugary foods with preservatives and additives.
- Take a vitamin D supplement, if necessary, and get out in the sunshine a bit more. This helps to build stronger bones and a healthy immune system.
- Take a probiotic supplement every day containing lacto-bacillus and bifidobacterium, to keep the gut flora strong and protected and the immune system supported. Try to take it first thing in the morning when the stomach is not too acidic. Eating live yoghurt with no added sugars is beneficial, or a fermented milk drink such as kefir. Also, eating a raw carrot before a meal is excellent for digestion, as this acts as a prebiotic that feeds the good bacteria more efficiently.
- Keep hydrated with plenty of filtered water throughout the day. Don't drink with meals though, so as not to dilute those essential digestive enzymes.
- Take exercise that you love and enjoy and that makes you feel invigorated and happy. This can be walking your dog or going to an exercise class.
- Try a meditation or yoga practice that allows you to clear your mind, stretching and releasing tension from your body, and try to take the time out and relaxation you need – even just 15 minutes each day to sit quietly and reconnect with yourself to see how you're feeling and to breathe deeply and consciously.
- Slow down and enjoy life. Try not to take problems from work to your home by finding a good work/home-life balance.
- See friends and family that you love who support you and make you laugh. This is important in sustaining your joy in life – that *joie de vivre*.

The History of Adaptogens

Adaptogen herbs work, as the name suggests, by helping the body adapt to life and, in particular, to the stresses of our environment. Adaptogens are a relatively new herbal grouping, and were first named by one of the Soviet Union's leading pharmacologists, Nikolai Lazarev, in the 1940s from the Latin word *adaptare*, meaning 'to adjust'.

Lazarev was asked by the Soviet government to help find a way to make the people of the USSR stronger and more resilient, especially their army and their workers, gymnasts and dancers, in the country's quest to dominate the West. They wanted to see improvement in their performance and overall stamina and Lazarev started to research scientifically the elite herbs used in traditional Chinese medicine. The results were so favourable that a whole research plan was started that spanned decades.

The boundaries are hard to define in classifying adaptogens. Many herbalists believe that to be classed as an adaptogen, the herb should not act on any one specific body organ but on the whole body system. Others believe the herb should have a direct effect on the hypothalamic–pituitary–adrenal axis (the HPA axis), which consists of these three endocrine glands and the complex interaction between these glands that regulates the way the body reacts to stress and works to allow the body to adapt effectively to these stressors.

Many are less concerned about defining a herb by whether or not its actions have a direct influence on the HPA axis, but more on whether it relieves nervous tension and supports the body's ability to cope with stress, increasing the body's overall health and vitality. This is definitely my stance on this group of adaptogen herbs.

The use of adaptogen herbs dates back thousands of years to ancient China and India, long before full understanding of how the body functioned. However, there was understanding of the interaction between an individual and their environment, and this energetic relationship between the two was regarded as being essential to good health. To find balance between our inner health and the environment around us encourages a state of wholeness and general good health.

Adaptogens are extraordinary, awe-inspiring herbs that can help the body maintain this homeostasis or equilibrium. They contain a wide range of botanical constituents that help our bodies cope, supporting the body so it doesn't suffer 'burnout'. These botanical constituents help to rebalance and deflect stress from the body by nourishing and stabilising the whole body system.

Prolonged stress can have a debilitating effect on our immune system, digestive health, endocrine and nervous system, and on general well-being. Managing and being able to deal with stress and its effects is the core of adaptogen herbs' action, when our bodies may just lack that vital force that is needed to drive these resources into action. I like to think of the herbs as support givers, providing a much-needed foundation when you're going through a particularly difficult time, or even when just feeling overwhelmed by the pressures of everyday living, by helping to increase much-needed resilience and stamina.

Stress is also ageing and in a society that is obsessed with looking young, working on the inside instead of just the outside is so important. Protecting and supporting our body's vitality is the key. Ageing well is not just about surviving to a ripe old age and trying to look younger than our years; it's about feeling well and youthful on the inside and not suffering ill health during this time. Healthy ageing should be our true goal when we look at our health.

Dr James Fries of the Stanford University School of Medicine asked why people acquire more chronic diseases as they age. He discovered that in youth we have a biological reserve of energy in our organs that we can draw on when confronted with stress or illness, but which returns to a baseline reserve level after use. As we age we lose energy from this organ reserve, and the rate at which we lose this determines how well we age.

Adaptogen herbs, along with healthy, positive lifestyle choices, including a compassionate, supportive and loving environment, can support this organ reserve and help us age in a graceful, healthful way, acquiring beauty and youthfulness on the inside as well as on the outside.

Adaptogens work in a non-specific way; they act generally on the whole body system but not on any one specific organ. They are non-toxic to the body and help in detoxifying the system. It's believed that most adaptogens contain high levels of anti-oxidants which help protect the body against cell damage, and they keep the pathways of elimination working at their optimal level. They help balance the whole body to achieve a healthful state – the perfect tonic to get you back on track after an illness, helping to build up your strength and vitality. And if you suffer from a long-standing chronic condition, they help to support the whole body system when it's feeling under pressure.

Adaptogens and You

The healing power of nature has been used through the centuries and we have extensive records of this use that has influenced the way we use plants today. The Egyptians were incredibly skilled in plant medicine and so much has been learnt from their surviving documentation, written on papyrus from about 1500 BC. The most famous of these sources is the Ebers Papyrus, a 110-metre scroll that documented their aware-ness of many diseases, including tumours. And around AD 60 a Greek physician, Dioscorides, wrote the five-volume *De Materia Medica*, which was probably the most influential work on medic-inal plants and their uses for the next 1,500 years.

The Egyptians ate garlic and onions to build up strength and vitality, to ease asthma and lung congestion and for a strong car-diovascular system. Herbs were steeped in wine or macerated in vinegars. They used aloe, basil, dill, liquorice, garlic and thyme and many other herbs, very much influencing how we use them today.

According to the World Health Organization, over 75 per cent of the world's population still depends directly on herbal plants for their basic health needs.

The Dalai Lama's *Paradox of Our Times* expresses the dilemma we face in our modern society as we have '*more knowledge but less judgement, more experts but more problems and more medicines but less wellness*'. The market has rows and rows of supplements, new fads and diets which can make it so difficult to know where to start or even which direction to take.

When I recommend a herbal remedy to a client I try to consider all aspects of their health and which herb will best support their needs. I always familiarise them with the herbs that I prescribe so they know what they're taking and how it's going to work in supporting their system, making them a knowledgeable and conscious participant in their own healing.

Superherbs will help support this, and the adaptogens in this book can be easily incorporated into your daily health programme.

How to Find Your Superherb

I've included twenty of my favourite, most accessible, primary adaptogen herbs in this book. You might think adaptogens such as turmeric or amla berries are not traditionally classed as herbs, and you would be right. Today the definitions have become blurred and amla is a fruit and turmeric is actually a spice. Spices are the root, bark, seed, flower and fruit of the plant, and herbs are the leafy part. There are some plants that herbalists use as both herbs and spices and they are classed as both, however all fall under the classification of herbal medicine.

For each herb I have listed my favourite uses, facts about its habitat, family, individual properties, folklore and history so you can understand each adaptogen, making them more accessible and allowing you to form your own relationship with them. I've included ten of my favourite ways to use each of them to inspire you to feel confident enough to incorporate these adaptogens into your daily life, with a few recipes, formulas, tonics, tinctures, infusions, beauty tonics, poultices, smoothies, juices and elixirs. These are simply suggestions and as you feel more comfortable with each herb, you can experiment with your own!

The adaptogens are listed alphabetically to make it easy for you to find the information. On page 263 I have listed my favourite stockists, but feel free to find your own reliable source.

Generally I would try and find stockists that provide wildcrafted, organic produce.

The best way to use this book is to familiarise yourself with each adaptogen herb and find the ones that resonate the most with you, rather than just one or two herbs and their actions – that way you'll find the one that's best suited to your individual needs.

An Important Note
Before You Get Started

Generally speaking, adaptogens are safe to use over a period of time with no significant side effects or contraindications, but my advice would be to avoid this group of herbs if pregnant or breastfeeding, and always to seek the advice of a herbalist or qualified naturopath if you have a chronic illness or feel unsure of what to take. *If you are currently taking prescription medication you should consult your physician or a qualified naturopathic doctor to ensure that there are no adverse interactions.*

I don't believe that this body of herbs called adaptogens is here to help us push beyond our own natural abilities to cope with the negatives life throws at us. Instead, we should listen to our bodies when they're telling us to slow down and to allow these nourishing herbs to replenish and support, rather than to push us to complete mental and physical exhaustion. They shouldn't be seen as a replacement for sleep, good nutrition or a much-needed life change when things are not working well for you.

They are not a quick fix; nor will one herb work for everyone. Herbs affect everyone in different ways; there's not one herbal remedy that suits everyone. These herbs are not miracle workers. They must be used in conjunction with your own positive individual lifestyle choices and should also be taken every day for a few months for the body to properly recognise and respond and utilise the herb in the most constructive way. This group of herbs in general can be taken safely over a long period of time.

As with any herbal remedy, I'd recommend starting off slowly and increasing the dosage as you become more familiar with its effects on your body system.

Now on to the herbs – I hope you enjoy!

SUPER
HERBS

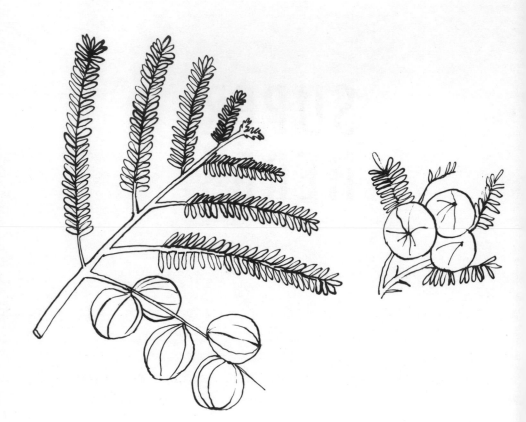

Amla

Emblica officinalis

Native to: India and Southeast Asia

My favourite uses: improving circulation, anaemia, liver tonic, high cholesterol and digestive weakness

Amla's Western name is Indian gooseberry as it looks very similar to the European gooseberry. In Hindi it is known as *amalka*, meaning 'the sustainer', and in Ayurveda it's known as *dhatri*, which means 'mother' or 'nurse'.

Amla is an evergreen tree belonging to the spurge family. It is native to and very common in India and southeast Asia. It grows up to 18 metres in height and its oblong leaves are small, slender and leathery; their fragrance is fresh and lemony. The astringent acidic fleshy fruit can also be sweet tasting, and only grows seven years after planting. They are ready for picking in abundance in the months from January to April.

The fruit is round and greenish in colour when unripe but then turns more yellow on ripening with six distinguishing vertical stripes around its diameter. Only the fully ripe fruit is used in Ayurvedic preparations.

This herbal food is revered in India as a 'super fruit' and 'divine medicine' and has been worshipped as the Earth Mother because of its nourishing, protective and cleansing properties, the fruit being used as a symbol of spiritual truth.

Amla has been used in Ayurvedic medicine for various ailments from headache to diarrhoea and is one of the ingredients in the Ayurvedic herbal formula known as Triphala, which is mainly used as a bowel tonic.

Traditionally all the parts of the tree can be used medicinally: the sap is applied topically on sores and the leaves used to make an eye wash. It can be used internally for indigestion and diarrhoea, with the flowers being used as a mild laxative, but it's the fruit that I'd like to bring to your attention here.

It is believed to be an antioxidant, anti-ulcer, anti-tumour, antidiabetic and antibacterial, as well as a cardio and liver protector with its ability to lower blood lipids.

According to Hindu legend, the amla tree's beginnings were from the tears of the goddesses Lakshmi and Parvati, whose tears of joy fell to Earth when they decided to worship Lord Shiva and Lord Vishnu in a new form.

For centuries it has been used every day as a *rasayana*, meaning 'path of essence' or a way of maintaining a healthy life physically, mentally and spiritually. There are are two types of *rasayana*: preventative and curative, and amla is both; a rejuvenating herbal food to enhance the body's vital energy, restoring its overall health with the belief in a long, youthful life.

How Amla Can Benefit You

Amla is sourly pungent and very bitter but, unusually, it has an unexpected sweet after-taste. In Ayurvedic medicine this has a cooling effect on the whole body system, which makes it a good liver tonic and excellent for those who retain heat or suffer from chronic inflammation.

The fruit is exceptionally high in antioxidant molecules including polyphenols, vitamin C, flavonoids, tannins and gallic acids, making this a super fruit with super free-radical scavenging abilities that is mostly unknown outside India ... but I believe this is all going to change!

Mind

Amla is nurturing for the heart and the blood vessels, keeping the body's circulatory system nourished and vibrant. This also has a positive effect on brain function, assisting with concentration and memory.

Body

Amla has been known traditionally over the centuries as one of the best rejuvenating adaptogen herbs, used to relieve and prevent circulatory, digestive and respiratory illnesses and helping to clear the lungs of chronic phlegm.

It is used for keeping the fire in the belly strong by stimulating the digestive enzymes with its bitter taste so that the whole digestive system is supported and working at its optimum, which is absolutely essential for good health.

The fruit has a high vitamin C content which helps to improve the absorption and assimilation of other nutrients from foods, such as iron and calcium. This makes it a good remedy for anaemia and in caring for bones and teeth. It is also strengthening to the eyes and assists in alleviating any ophthalmic problems, especially those associated with ageing.

Amla also supports and regenerates the body's connective tissues, making it a beneficial herb for those suffering from autoimmune diseases such as rheumatoid arthritis and in helping prevent other age-related degenerative illnesses.

There are studies that show amla may also help in the prevention of cancer, with its beneficial free-radical scavenging effects, but amla's strong antioxidant effects may interfere with chemotherapy and radiation treatments, so please check with your specialist before using.

This superherb is a powerful antioxidant and helps to support immune function, assisting the body's disease resistance and preventing infection. These antioxidants will also have a positive effect in boosting fertility in both men and women.

There has been much research into using amla for liver damage. The tannoid and flavonoid constituents in amla protect the liver, especially where there has been alcohol damage, and help to improve the liver's filtration system.

Research has confirmed that this small bitter fruit improves HDL, high density lipoprotein, the protective cholesterol and lowers LDL, low density lipoprotein or 'bad' cholesterol, in diabetic patients.

Beauty and Spirit

The most natural way to get a daily dose of vitamin D is to expose your unprotected skin to the sun and its UVB rays. You don't need to stay in the sun for long and you don't need to tan to get vitamin D into your system. Unfortunately a lot of us, including myself, have exposed our skin to a lot more sun than it needed!

Amla's high antioxidant content extends to protecting the collagen of the skin from the ultra-violet rays of the sun which are known to damage skin cells. UVB rays are responsible for sunburn, but UVA penetrates the deep layers of the skin and causes the signs of ageing.

Ten Ways with Amla

1. Grow Your Own

Most adaptogens have to adapt to extreme environments in order to survive and the amla tree is no exception. It is tough and resistant and can withstand snowfall and the extreme heat of the summer. It doesn't like frost though, so care should be taken to wrap your growing amla with protective materials such as hessian and straw or bubble-wrap at its base.

It may take five to seven years to bear fruit but it's worth the wait for this golden investment!

2. An Amla a Day . . .

Try eating onc amla berry a day to reap the health benefits of this superherb. A pinch of salt helps your palate adjust to the sour taste, and a sip of water makes the fruit super sweet. Amazing but true!

I have a delivery from an online Indian herb and spice company. See page 263 for my favourite stockists. Look for firm yellow fruit; they should stay fresh for around four or five days.

3. Amla and Ginger Juice for Longevity

This ginger and amla juice gets the digestive juices fired up, so it is best drunk in the morning on an empty stomach.

5 fresh amla, chopped and deseeded
4 sprigs of curry leaves
3–5cm piece of fresh ginger, peeled
1 teaspoon of Himalayan salt to counteract the sourness of the
  amla and for detoxifying
2 cups of water

Place everything in a blender except the water and blend till everything is mixed and the amla is smooth. Add the water and blend again. Strain the juice and drink.

4. Refreshing Amla Smoothie

This cooling smoothie is great at any time of day and will help you top up your daily fruit and veggie allowance.

1 cup of spinach
1 cup of blueberries
1 cup of pea shoots
3 cups of almond milk
1 tablespoon of coconut oil
2 teaspoons of amla powder (see page 263 for stockists) or 2
  fresh amla, cut into small pieces
3 teaspoons of bee pollen

Put the spinach, blueberries, pea shoots, almond milk, coconut oil and, if using, fresh amla pieces into a blender. (If using amla powder add this with the bee pollen at the end.) Mix until smooth. Add the amla powder and bee pollen, stir and enjoy!

5. Ginger, Honey and Lemon Twist

The usual benefits of ginger, honey and lemon with hot water with the added boost of amla to add that extra medicinal hit to get you back on your feet after a cold or tummy upset.

4 amla
5cm piece of ginger, peeled
1 cup of hot boiling water
1 tablespoon of honey

Juice of 1 lemon
1 teaspoon of cinnamon
1 teaspoon of dried dandelion root

Chop the amla and the ginger into thin slices and place in a saucepan. Add the hot water, bring to the boil and simmer for 15–20 minutes.

Take off the heat, add the honey, lemon juice, cinnamon and dandelion root and stir. Pour into a cup, allowing the amla and ginger to settle at the bottom, and then enjoy this balancing healing drink.

6. Nourishing Amla Chutney

This chutney is a delicious way of adding amla to your diet.

5 fresh amla
4 cloves of garlic
2 green chillies
Sea salt
1 tablespoon of oil
2 teaspoons of mustard seeds
2 teaspoons of cumin seeds
A few curry leaves
2 teaspoons of turmeric powder
Handful of fresh coriander, chopped

First wash the amla and cut into small pieces. Put the amla, garlic, chillies and salt into a blender and mix until they form a paste. Add a little water if necessary to make it less dry. Put the paste into a bowl.

Heat a little oil in a frying pan and add the mustard seeds, cumin seeds, curry leaves and turmeric powder and fry for a

minute, stirring over the heat until the mustard seeds start popping and the ingredients mix together.

Turn off the heat and add the amla paste to the spices in the
pan and mix well.

Add the chopped coriander leaves and you have a delicious
nutritious chutney.

7. Refreshing Spicy Chutney

This should last in the fridge for up to 3 days.

3 fresh amla
1 bunch of coriander leaves, chopped
½ fresh green chilli, deseeded and chopped
Juice of 1 lime
Himalayan salt to taste

Cut the flesh of the amla off the seed and discard the seeds. Add
everything to a blender and pulse until all the ingredients are
mixed. Add enough water little by little to the mixture, giving a
little pulse after each addition, to form a paste. Add salt to taste.

Transfer to a dish and enjoy.

8. Easy Amla Jam

Use this tasty jam as a spread or add to porridge or yoghurt. Keep
in a sterilised jar in the fridge for 3–4 months.

10 medium-sized fresh amla
1 cup of coconut sugar
3 teaspoons of cinnamon
Juice of half a fresh lemon

Place the fruit whole in a saucepan, cover with water and put a lid on. Simmer for 15 minutes.

Take off the heat and strain. When cooled remove the seeds and discard them, chop up the fruit and place in a saucepan over a medium heat.

Add the coconut sugar and cinnamon and stir continuously, adding another cup of water slowly as you stir for another 10 minutes.

Take off the heat and mash with a potato masher or the back of a spoon.

Add the juice of the half lemon and place back on the heat for 10 minutes or until the consistency is mushy but not too watery as then it won't keep (but not too thick either as it'll become too hard).

Remove from the heat, allow to cool and store in a sterilised jar or airtight container.

9. Amla Honey

This takes a lot of honey to make but it can be used continuously to make as much amla honey as you like, so it starts a kind of amla honey production line. Spread on toast or add to your herbal infusion.

8 fresh medium–large amla
A pot of good quality organic thick honey
2 sterilised airtight glass jars, larger than the honey jar

Wash the amla and cut into thin slices around the seeds; throw the seeds away. Place the amla pieces in a clean jar and pour over the honey to completely cover the fruit.

Place the honey-and-amla jar in the sun for 4–6 days, shaking the jar each day. The honey will start to thin as the amla loses moisture; this takes about 4 days.

Take another clean sterilised glass jar and place the original amla pieces into this jar. Pour in fresh honey to cover all the amla fruit again. (The original batch of honey can be used to make another jar of amla honey.) Cover and store for up to three weeks, until the amla pieces are soft.

You can take the honey daily. It is a deliciously sweet way to get the daily health benefits of amla.

10. Amla and Rose Face Mask

Amla's high antioxidant constituents make a wonderful anti-ageing face mask, and rose helps to soothe, tone and cool tired skin.

1 tablespoon of amla powder
1 tablespoon of rose water

Mix the amla powder with the rose water and spread over a clean face with clean fingers. Leave on for 15–30 minutes before rinsing off with a clean cloth and warm water.

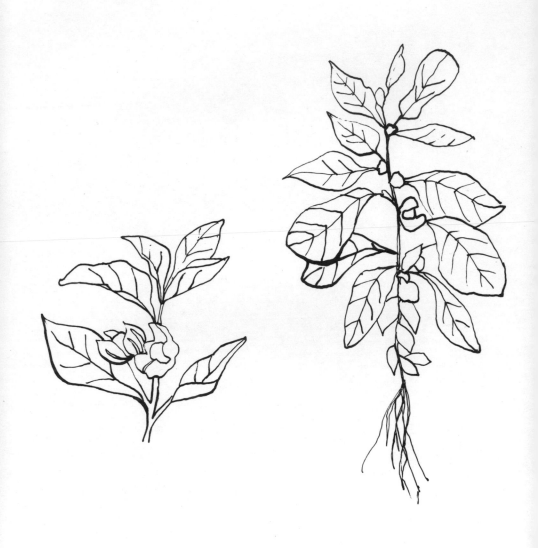

Ashwagandha

Withania somnifera

Native to: warm climates such as the Mediterranean, Africa, India and the Far East

My favourite uses: helps when there's a general lack of energy and vitality, to reduce stress, feelings of fatigue, or when there's difficulty focusing and concentrating

Ashwagandha is a plump woody shrub that is one of the tomato and nightshade family (Solanacaea). It has oval leaves, yellow flowers and small red fruit the size of raisins. It typically grows in warm climates around the world from the Med and Africa, to India and the Far East. The root is the part that is mainly used medicinally even though the leaves and fruit also have therapeutic properties. The root is dug up carefully when the whole shrub matures and then this root is dried and made into a powder or sliced to make a decoction – a method of extracting the medicinal contents of your herb by boiling it in water (this works best with roots and rhizomes) – or tincturing. This is a method of using alcohol as a solvent to extract the herb's medicinal properties.

This is an ancient Ayurvedic herb. Ayurvedic medicine is one of the oldest holistic healing methods, originating in India over 3,000 years ago, and ashwagandha is considered one of its most revered and powerful primary adaptogens. It is classified in Ayurveda as a *rasayana*, which means a herb known to promote both physical and mental health. It also has a dual action in both energising and calming the body, depending on its needs. It is often referred to as Indian ginseng because of its rejuvenating and anti-stress effects on the body, but botanically these herbs are not related.

The name in Sanskrit means 'the smell of a horse', which most probably relates to its strength and vigour – and the belief that anyone taking this herb will gain stallion-like qualities. Its botanical family name *somnifera* means 'restful sleep', suggesting its adaptogenic effects in its ability to calm and restore the body.

How Ashwagandha Can Benefit You

My favourite uses of ashwagandha include helping with anxiety, stress, lack of energy, inflammation, low sexual libido, difficulty concentrating and focusing. If you're feeling a general lack of enthusiasm, anxious, overwhelmed and exhausted by life and in need of vitality and more energy, then this is a perfect remedy.

Ashwagandha contains many useful plant constituents, including alkaloids, withanolides and fatty acids, which all have anti-inflammatory, antioxidant, anti-stress and immune-system enhancing properties. It works with a wide range of conditions, including anxiety, nervous exhaustion, insomnia, arthritis, asthma and psoriasis.

Mind

In India ashwagandha is known as the go-to herb when learning or when suffering from poor concentration and brain fog, helping with mental clarity. The high antioxidant content of ashwagandha has been seen to be beneficial in having a positive effect on brain function in treating the symptoms of dementia and Alzheimer's disease, such as memory loss, misplacing belongings and disorientation.

There are many tests being done on the leaves of ashwagandha as there is a compound found in the leaves called glycol that has been found to naturally induce sleep, and may be beneficial to those who suffer from insomnia.

Body

Ashwagandha helps to energise the body, but rather than also jangling and stimulating the mind it has a soothing, calming effect, helping to support you when modern life, work or multitasking is putting you under extra strain.

It is a rich source of iron, so it is a good remedy for treating anaemia and its symptoms of general fatigue, weakness and dizziness. Ashwagandha is also believed to support the thyroid and is seen to be helpful with the exhausting symptoms of hypothyroidism.

This incredible herb has been found to enhance chemotherapy and radiation therapy while reducing the toxic effects these treatments can have on the body's organs. It also acts as a tonic, helping to improve the body's overall recovery. A lot more research needs to be done, though, before ashwagandha is used alongside conventional chemo and radiation therapy. If you are suffering from cancer, please have a discussion with your oncologist and chemo pharmacist before embarking on any herbal or nutritional remedies.

Ashwagandha has been used for centuries as a sexual restorative and aphrodisiac, helping those with a lowered sexual libido. There are many reasons for a lowered libido but the most common are hormonal imbalances, impaired immunity and stress. It is also a good herb for strengthening the female reproductive system and for male infertility or impotence.

Where there's chronic, debilitating upper respiratory tract diseases such as emphysema, asthma and TB, ashwagandha is a herb to consider.

Ashwagandha eases muscle spasm and tension and acts as a central nervous system relaxant, which is helpful in many chronic conditions such as fibromyalgia. This condition is believed to be brought on by physical or emotional stress and can cause many debilitating symptoms including a sensitivity to pain, forgetfulness, muscle stiffness and digestive problems. This superherb's ability to nurture the nervous system also helps to ease anxiety and the feeling of being completely overwhelmed and 'stressed out' – a term used so often that it has lost its real meaning.

Beauty and Spirit

In animal studies, ashwagandha has been found to be as effective as conventional medicinal hydrocortisone in calming inflammation and soothing irritated skin.

Ashwagandha's strong anti-inflammatory properties work well in relieving the symptoms of arthritic and rheumatic conditions such as pain, stiffness and swelling.

The high levels of antioxidants within this herb help to keep the negative degenerative side effects of ageing at bay, and it has also been used with great success by athletes who put their bodies under great physical stress, helping with metabolism and vitality and enhancing their natural stamina.

Ten Ways with Ashwagandha

Ashwagandha has a strong pungent taste when eaten and this bitter taste automatically stimulates the digestive enzymes, helping them to flow and thus improving the overall digestive process. This is why it's a good idea to take this herb in powdered form, by grinding the root in a coffee grinder so that it can be added to food. The taste may not be to your liking, so add herbs with flavour that can also support your digestion, such as ginger, cinnamon and cardamom.

1. Grow Your Own Ashwagandha

As a society we generally feel more comfortable buying something already prepared for us with instructions and a guarantee, but I'd like to challenge this by encouraging you to try and grow your very own ashwagandha plant. Not only is it a great way to familiarise yourself with ashwagandha but it is also enjoyable and relaxing. Why not try growing all twenty herbs recommended in this book?

Ashwagandha is unique as an adaptogen herb as it is very easy to cultivate. It is from the nightshade family and is very similar and as easy to propagate as tomatoes, which belong to the same family.

Around three weeks before Spring officially gets under way, on a frost-free, warmish day, sow seeds bought from a reputable nursery in seed trays or in individual small flowerpots, placing two or three seeds in each pot, covering with a thin layer of seed compost and gently firming it over the seeds. Water using a mister or gently drizzle water over the top and keep them indoors until the seeds germinate. This will probably take around two to three weeks.

When the weather gets warmer and Spring is definitely here

with no chance of frost, transplant the seeds to a sunny spot in the garden. In Autumn the small berries will start to ripen to an orangey red.

After around a year the root should be mature enough for medicinal use. Pull up the plant and cut off the root to dry. Wash it carefully first and place it in a dark, warm, dry place for a few weeks. When dry, the root can be chopped and used.

2. Soothing Milk Drink

Traditionally ashwagandha was added as a powder to warm milk with honey, especially for stress and insomnia. There are many types of non-dairy milk that you can use if you'd prefer. My personal preference is almond milk, which works well heated, or soya milk.

1 cup of preferred choice of milk
2 teaspoons of ashwagandha powder

Gently simmer the milk and root powder, whisking to blend the two together. You can add honey for sweetness, preferably Manuka honey for its digestive system-supporting properties, and a sprinkling of cardamom and/or allspice for their digestive support and warming flavours.

To help you unwind before bed sip this half an hour before-hand, and take it regularly like this for a few months so that your body starts to assimilate the medicinal calming benefits.

Ashwagandha was also added to ghee, a clarified butter rich in nutrients and beneficial to the digestive tract.

3. Thyme and Ashwagandha Honey Pot

Try adding thyme to this infused honey, which increases its antibacterial and antiviral properties. It will also mask some of the pungent flavour of the ashwagandha. The honey will last for several months stored in a cool dry place.

A jar of good quality honey
5 teaspoons of ashwagandha powder
Chopped thyme (optional)

Mix the honey and ashwagandha in a sterilised honey jar. Add the chopped thyme, if you like. Spread the honey on any of your favourites such as toast or a sliced apple, or even use it to sweeten your herbal infusions.

4. Hemp Seed Butter or Nut Butters with Ashwagandha

Adding ashwagandha's adaptogen benefits to omega-rich nut butters is another easy way to add the power of this herb to your diet. This will keep for up to three months.

A jar of seed or nut butter – my favourite is almond
5 teaspoons of unsweetened desiccated coconut to add a little
  extra flavour
5 teaspoons of ashwagandha powder

Mix these three ingredients together in a sterilised jar and add to toast or fruit at breakfast, or for a delicious, nutritious, overall holistic snack.

5. Raw Cinnamon and Ashwagandha Chocolate

This is a delicious, energising sweet treat with no refined sugars. You can make some for family and friends, too! It will keep in your fridge for up to a week.

5 teaspoons of ashwagandha powder
½ cup of raw cocoa powder
1 teaspoon of cinnamon powder
1 teaspoon of ground cardamom
½ teaspoon of salt
½ cup of coconut sugar
½ cup of coconut butter
½ cup of almond butter

Mix all the ingredients together. Place in a chocolate mould or on greaseproof paper and put in the freezer to set.

6. Ashwagandha Latte

This is a fantastic substitute for caffeinated drinks and will give you more consistent energy and enhance a positive mood.

2 cups of almond milk
2 teaspoons of ashwagandha powder
1 teaspoon of ground cardamom
1 dessertspoon of good honey
Pinch of Himalayan salt

Heat the milk and the ashwagandha powder in a saucepan over a low heat until the milk reduces a little. This infuses the ashwagandhda into the milk.

Add the ground cardamom to the honey and stir into your hot latte. Add a pinch of Himalayan salt to taste.

7. Energising and Balancing Ayurvedic Smoothie

A delicious warming Ayurvedic smoothie for an early morning pick-me-up and energy balancer.

1 teaspoon of cinnamon powder
1 teaspoon of turmeric powder
1 teaspoon of ashwagandha powder
1 teaspoon of Holy Basil/tulsi (see page 131)
3 cups of nut or cows' milk
1 banana
½ cup of oats
1 tablespoon of coconut oil

Blend all the ingredients together for a positive early start to your day.

8. Transformational Breakfast Topper

I find it really handy to have a jar of tasty additions to add to my morning porridge and cereal to give it that extra nutritious and detoxifying bite. This should keep for four weeks in an airtight jar.

1 tablespoon of bee pollen
1 tablespoon of chia seeds
1 tablespoon of roughly chopped dates
1 tablespoon of toasted seasame seeds
1 tablespoon of flax seeds
5 teaspoons of ashwagandha powder
5 teaspoons of cacao powder
5 teaspoons of astragalus powder (see page 29)

Add all the ingredients to an airtight jar, put the lid on and give it a shake. Keep in the cupboard as a transformational breakfast topper.

9. Decoction of Ashwagandha

The word 'decoct' means to extract the essence from a hard material through boiling or heating. A decoction is a concentrated liquid obtained through boiling and simmering a hard woody herb or root in water to allow the soluble medicinal properties to be transferred from the root into the water as just a simple infusion with these wouldn't be enough.

In order to do this you need to use a glass and an earthenware or enamelled saucepan – *please do not use aluminium as this can leach into the water*.

Chop the ashwagandha root so that its medicinal properties mix with the water. Pour a few cups of cold filtered water into a saucepan with 1 teaspoon of the dried root. (You can double or triple the amounts if desired and then reheat the liquid when needed during the day.)

Cover the pan, bring to the boil and then simmer for 15–20 minutes. Turn off the heat and strain the liquid or leave it on the stove until it is a drinkable temperature. Let the root naturally settle at the bottom of the pan.

You may like the earthy taste, which will do wonders for your digestive system, or add a little good quality honey to taste.

A tincture is another way of taking ashwagandha but without the immediate digestive benefits. It does assimilate well within your system and often has a longer shelf life than tablets and powder, and is often easier if you're on the go.

Fluid extracts and tinctures

Fluid extracts and tinctures are concentrated liquid extracts of a herb, usually made with alcohol as a solvent (80–100 per cent proof such as vodka). You may choose to use 50 per cent of the alcohol by adding the tincture to boiling water, or you may prefer not to use alcohol at all: apple cider vinegar or vegetable glycerin are also effective solvents for all the medicinal goodness.

You can find good quality tinctures and fluid extracts of herbs at Neal's Yard Remedies and The Organic Herb Company (see page 263), but if you want to try your hand at tincturing yourself here's how.

For dried roots such as ashwagandha, finely chop with a good knife or coffee grinder. Use enough to fill your chosen sterilised dry jar a quarter full and place the chopped root or powder in the bottom of the jar.

Pour over the alcohol to the very top of the jar, covering the herbs completely. Leave this to soften or macerate over 4–6 weeks at room temperature, gently shaking the jar daily to allow the herb to mix with the alcohol.

Strain the herbs from the liquid using muslin or a fine strainer, preserving the tincture in a new bottle, and label and date it so everyone knows what is in there and when it was made. An amber bottle is preferable as this helps to preserve the medicinal properties by keeping out the light.

A fluid extract contains the same amount of herb and alcohol in a ratio of 1:1. It's often three to four times stronger than a tincture.

Keep in mind that tinctures and fluid extracts made with alcohol have a warming effect on the system that will not be beneficial when treating conditions that need cooling, such as inflammation.

10. Balm for Arthritic Joints

This soothing balm will help ease inflammation and painful joints. Rub into the fingertips and massage on to the affected area.

75ml of almond oil
25g of shea butter
5g of beeswax
3ml of vitamin E oil
1 teaspoon of cayenne pepper
4 teaspoons of ashwagandha powder
8 drops of ginger essential oil
A few small jars

A bain-marie is a stainless steel or enamel bowl which sits over a saucepan that is a quarter-full of boiling water, allowing the steam rather than the water to heat the bowl, and dissolve and warm the ingredients gently.

Add the above ingredients, except the ginger essential oil, to the bain-marie and simmer gently until the beewax has dissolved and all the ingredients have mixed together.

Add the ginger essential oil, give it a quick stir and then take off the heat. Pour the mixture into small jars with lids and allow to cool.

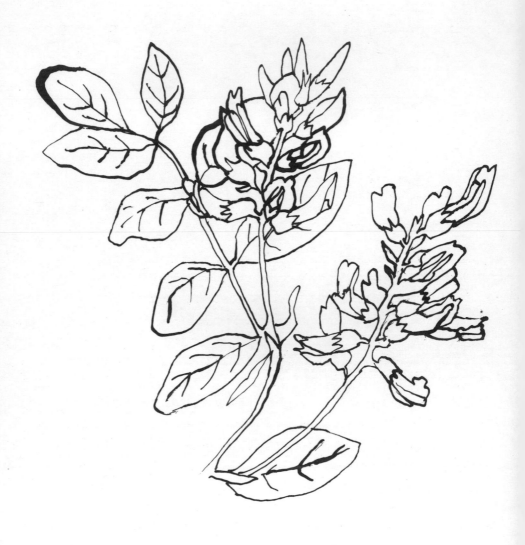

Astragalus

Astragalus membranaceus

Native to: China and Siberia

My favourite uses: to build up the immune system, for those depleted after a long illness, lethargy, chronic chest complaints and exhaustion, to lift and protect a deflated spirit, for those suffering from fear

Astragalus is also known as milk-vetch root or *ogi* in Japanese and belongs to the bean and pea family. This pretty plant with its delicate pink-hued flowers can reach about 40cm in height and produces hairy stems and leaves that have soft, long and oval fern-like fronds. It loves a sandy soil with lots of sunshine and is generally found across China, Siberia and Mongolia where it is grown for its medicinal properties and is usually harvested after about four years, in the spring.

This herb is a primary adaptogen in Chinese medicine and is known as *huang-qi*, meaning 'yellow energy' or 'yellow leader', most probably because of the root colour when dried. It is considered one of the most important herbs in traditional Chinese medicine (TCM), used as a tonic to strengthen *qi*, our vital energy, and our defensive *qi* which works to protect our bodies from outside influences that are cold and damp, supporting the immune system, treating colds, respiratory disorders, fatigue and increasing our energy levels.

Astragalus is known to support heart and liver function, and it also works to enhance the spleen, an abdominal organ which stores our blood and any excess red blood cells. The spleen is also an important part of the immune system. There was a time when allopathic doctors thought the spleen was not essential to health, like the appendix, but it is now known that people without a spleen run a greater risk of infection than those who have one. (In TCM yellow is the colour associated with the spleen.)

How Astragalus Can Benefit You

Astragalus contains many healing constituents such as poly-saccharides and astragaloids, and is a rich source of potassium, magnesium and selenium, essential minerals that work together for a heathy heart and nervous system.

There are no known side effects when using this herb and it is believed to be safe for the elderly and young alike, and for those who are really unwell and are unable to tolerate many remedies.

It really does taste delicious – a little sweet and earthy. This isn't just my opinion. I've always taken this herb myself and I've given it to my children when they've had the flu or are feeling run down and exhausted; this is one of the few herbs that they don't ever complain about when I pop a few drops of fluid extract in their water or add the root to soups and casseroles.

I believe astragalus can help us with positive ageing, as a tonic adaptogen for the elderly to support the whole body system. Astragalus supports digestion, the urinary system, the heart and the nervous system, which can all suffer as we get older; for these reasons alone it is one of my favourite herbs.

Mind

This herb lifts you up when you're exhausted and depressed, especially if the body and mind's vital energy is depleted due to illness. I recommend astragalus to strengthen not just the mind but also the spirit. I tell my patients to think of this herb as a protective shield or a cloak around them, keeping their immune system strong and their vital energy alive.

Body

Astragalus is a herb that's recommended for spleen deficiency symptoms such as tiredness and lack of appetite. I use this herb as an energising tonic to strengthen and stimulate the immune system, especially after an illness when there's generally poor and weakened health.

Astragalus helps to prevent and treat infections, a chronic illness or recurring virus, especially chest infections. It acts as a tonic for the lungs, especially in chronic conditions such as asthma, and is particularly good after an infection of the lungs.

As mentioned, astragalus works well with those suffering from chronic illness, helping to reduce inflammation, balancing blood sugars and the hormonal system.

It helps the body attain its optimum potential, overcome stress and enhances the immune system by stimulating white blood cell production. It's also a good go-to remedy when suffering from flu or the common cold.

As a kidney tonic, it helps to flush out the system. It works as a mild diuretic and therefore improves the kidney's *qi*, which in turn improves the body's overall energy levels.

Astragalus is believed to be beneficial to the cardiovascular system, working as a heart protector, strengthening and improving circulation and in some cases having a blood-thinning effect, helping to reduce blood clotting.

There needs to be more clinical trials to evaluate the effect of astragalus on diabetes but there is evidence that it may be able to improve blood sugar levels.

Athletes have found that astragalus helps to increase their strength and stamina. It helps in the uptake of oxygen, which increases endurance, and athletes have also found the herb reduces their recovery time.

Beauty and Spirit

Astragalus is considered a wonderful remedy for persistent skin blemishes, and for more serious skin conditions such as ulcers or infections that recur and do not heal.

It will also help support a child with chicken pox, shortening the longevity and severity of the illness.

Ten Ways with Astragalus

The root of astragalus is easy to obtain from reputable health-food stores or online. The dried flat root looks a lot like a doctor's tongue suppressor.

1. Chew the Sticks

Chewing on the dried astragalus root is surprisingly tasty as well as beneficial. And very easy to do at any time of day!

2. Banana Smoothie

I make this when I need something nourishing and comforting.

1 medium-sized avocado, peeled and stoned
1 banana
½ cup of hemp powder
1½ cups of almond milk
Pinch of Himalayan salt
½ tablespoon of freeze-dried rose hip powder
2 teaspoons of astragalus powder

Add everything to a blender and pulse until mixed, and then drink.

3. Green Juice

This green juice is a perfect way to kick-start your morning and get your veggies in early.

A handful of kale
A whole (unwaxed) lemon with the skin on
A handful of watercress
A handful of baby spinach
1 teaspoon of astragalus powder
1 teaspoon of bee pollen.

Wash the veggie leaves and lemon and add to your juicer. Pour into a cup or container and stir in the astragalus powder and bee pollen.

4. Rev Up Your Porridge

Mix these powdered adaptogens into your porridge oats for support, nourishment and balance throughout the day.

1 teaspoon of astragalus
1 teaspoon of Siberian ginseng (see page 237)
1 teaspoon of rhodiola (see page 195)
1 teaspoon of linseed
4 teaspoons of good quality honey

Mix the above ingredients into a paste and stir into your freshly made porridge.

5. Astragalus and Dried Fruit Breakfast Ball

This gives consistent energy and support throughout the day.

½ cup of raisins
½ cup of dried apricots
½ cup of dried mango
3 tablespoons of almond butter
1 tablespoon of dried ground almonds
4 teaspoons of powdered astragalus
1 cup of dried shredded coconut

Blend or pulse all the ingredients apart from the shredded coconut in a blender. Be sure your hands are clean and then place a dessertspoonful of the mixture in your palm and roll into a ball. Sprinkle on the dried shredded coconut and you have a coconut-covered breakfast ball!

To store, place on a tray sprinkled with rice flour (to stop the balls sticking), and put in the fridge, where they should last around a week.

6. Astragalus and Chicken Broth

This is a great broth to prepare when feeling poorly with a cold or flu.

Oil for frying
4 spring onions, chopped
2 cloves of garlic, crushed
2 red chillies
4 organic chicken thighs and legs on the bone
1 litre chicken stock
2 dried astragalus roots
100g of kale, chopped
A handful of parsley, chopped
A sprig of thyme
A few mint leaves

Pour a little oil into a flameproof casserole dish and fry the spring onions and garlic on a medium heat till soft and a little golden.

Add the chillies and the chicken and fry until the chicken skin is golden. Pour in the chicken stock, add the astragalus and stir, and then place in a preheated oven for an hour with the lid on at 170°C/gas mark 3.

Take the casserole out after an hour and place back on the hob on a low heat and add the kale until this softens a little. Take off the heat, add all the herbs and serve.

7. Bone Broth with Astragalus

My mum used to prepare this as stock and swore by its health benefits. This is perfect to prepare and then have on hand to add to different dishes to give an immune-enhancing boost, or you can heat up a bowl of this broth when convalescing or exhausted, or just to improve your overall radiant health and skin.

Makes about 3 litres

3kg of organic (if possible) beef bones
3 cloves of garlic, roughly chopped
3 sticks of celery, roughly chopped
3 carrots, roughly chopped
2 large leeks, roughly chopped
¾ black peppercorns
1 tablespoon of apple cider
Sage leaves
Bay leaves
2 dried astragalus roots

Place the bones in a large stainless-steel cooking pot. Add the rest of the ingredients and enough water to cover to about 2.5cm deep. Bring to the boil, then reduce the heat and simmer with the lid on for a good 24 hours. Take off the heat and strain, then leave to cool and store.

8. Astragalus Decoction

This is a delicious, supportive warming beverage. I find it doesn't need any other herbs or sweetness such as honey but give it a try and see what you think.

Cut up the sliced dried astragalus root and add to two cups of filtered cold water in a flameproof glass, enamel or earthenware pot. Cover and bring to the boil. Then let it simmer for 15–20 minutes.

Let this cool on the stove to drinking temperature, which allows the root to sink to the bottom of the pan (or strain the root off with a tea strainer) and drink 2–3 times daily.

9. Astragalus Fluid Extract or Tincture

It's easy to break up the roots of astragalus by finely chopping them, using a good knife. Use enough to fill your chosen sterilised dry jar a quarter-full and then pour over the alcohol to the very top of the jar, covering the astragalus completely.

Leave this to macerate over 4–6 weeks at room temperature, gently shaking the jar daily to allow the herb to mix with the alcohol.

Strain the herb from the liquid using muslin or a fine strainer, preserving the tincture in a new bottle, labelled and dated so that everyone knows what is in there and when it was made. An amber bottle is preferable as this helps to preserve the medicinal properties.

10. Astragalus Antioxidant Mask

This mask is astringent and a perfect remedy for using on the skin when it is particularly greasy and problematic and in need of a deep detox.

2 teaspoons of astragalus powder
1 tablespoon of aloe vera gel
1 tablespoon of green clay
1 dessertspoon of rose hip oil
5 drops of clary sage essential oil

Mix all the ingredients together and apply immediately to clean, dry skin; leave on for 15 minutes. Rinse well with a clean cloth and warm water.

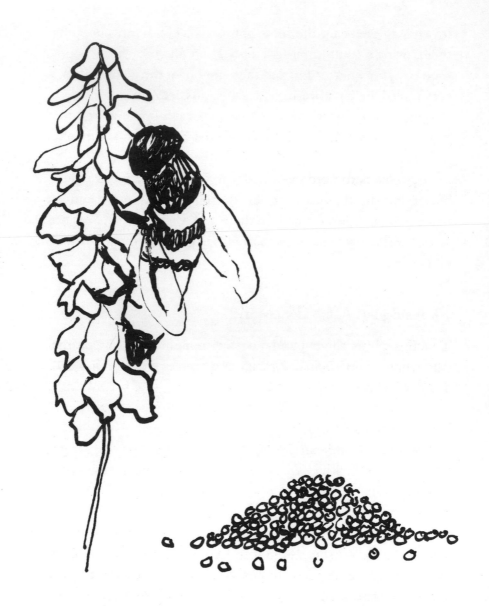

Bee Pollen and Propolis

Native to: found globally

My favourite uses: for detoxing, protection from environmental stressors, as an anti-ageing skin tonic, immune-system stimulant

Pollen is one of the many medicinal products of our incredible honeybee, *Apis mellifera*. For the last few years it has been a well-recorded super food and tried and tested by many celebrities, such as Victoria Beckham who attributes her graceful ageing to this little golden ball produced by the bee.

I admire all the healing medicinal foods our honeybees offer. As well as pollinating our food crops and wild plants they provide propolis ('bee glue'), honey (manuka being my favourite), royal jelly and bee pollen.

I try to use all of the honeybee's gifts: propolis is used in my healing balm, but something I use every morning is bee pollen. A fact that has me in awe and makes me honour and respect this daily ritual is that it takes one bee a whole month, working eight hours a day, to make just one teaspoon of this glorious bee pollen!

Bee pollen is derived from the male reproductive part of the flower and is made by the honeybee by packing or tamping the pollen down into the 'baskets' on their hind legs, making a pollen ball as they go from flower to flower. It is brought back to the hive to nourish the young bee colony, and for humans it's one of the most complete and nutritious foods available in nature, possessing 185 different nutritional ingredients. It also has more readily available protein in it than any animal source, making it invaluable to vegetarians.

This easily digestible alkaline food is rich in amino acid proteins, fatty acids – omega 3 and omega 6 – lecithin, B vitamins, vitamin C, vitamin D, vitamin E, vitamin K and folic acid. It is mineral rich with manganese, iron, phosphorus, copper, magnesium, zinc, calcium, potassium, sodium, boron, chromium, iodine and selenium. Pollen is also rich in antioxidants such as rutin, carotenoids and flavonoids, bioflavonoids and phytosterols, which are anti-inflammatory and anti-cancer.

Pollen also contains enzymes which support our digestive systems, carbohydrates for sustaining energy, and some magic secret bee ingredients that science still can't identify and may be its greatest attribute! Interestingly, humans have supposedly tried but failed to replicate the genius of bee pollen in a synthetic form.

The history of bee pollen's medicinal use, otherwise known as apitherapy, goes back to Egyptian times when bees were believed to be made from the tears of the sun god, Ra. The Greeks and Romans took raw honey containing bee pollen to help maintain health and longevity, and it was thought to be one of the ingredients in ambrosia – the food of the gods.

The biblical account from Genesis tells of pollen being on Earth before even man's existence, and our journey with the honeybee has probably been the longest.

There have been many reports on the benefits of bee pollen. One – whether fact or folklore – is from the 1940s from the

Russian biologist and botanist Nikolai Vasilevich Tsitsin. Tsitsin studied centenarians in the Caucasus mountains of Georgia, where he found many living to even one hundred and fifty! Wanting to know the common thread that each of these incredible 'oldies' had in common, he realised that they were mostly beekeepers who had a daily dose of the scrapings on the bottom of the beehive, containing all the unprocessed honey and pollen, while selling the clear, less nutritional honey on to the rest of the community.

At the Institute of Bee Culture in Paris the biologist and entomologist Remy Chauvin was fascinated by honeybees and, after observing them and their surrounding environment closely for decades, wrote many articles about them. He noted that bee pollen's constituents were antibiotic and, interestingly, bacteriostatic (capable of stopping the growth and reproduction of bacteria). This is different from a substance that is bactericidal, which kills bacteria such as salmonella and *E. coli* outright.

Propolis also has an incredible action which increases our resistance to disease. It is a mixture of resin from the buds and leaves of trees, pollen and beeswax, and was discovered by the bees thousands of years ago. It is collected on the bees' hind legs and used to build and fix hives. With its antimicrobial and antibiotic properties propolis keeps the hive sterile and free from bacteria, moulds and fungi.

Medical research has shown just how beneficial propolis is to us, with its antioxidant, anti-inflammatory and anti-cancer flavonoids. I use it in my own healing balm for wounds, especially for those with lowered immune systems who find it hard to heal, and with other skin conditions such as bacterial infections and burns. Russian scientists also believe propolis both enhances and potentiates other medicines such as antibiotics.

Internally try using propolis to support and boost the immune system against flu and chest infections and sore inflamed throats.

Propolis has mild analgesic properties which help to numb irritation as well as working its healing magic.

How Bee Pollen and Propolis Can Benefit You

Important note

Bee products such as propolis and pollen can have a negative effect on people with allergies to bee pollen or insect stings, with symptoms of dizziness and impaired breathing.

Consult your medical practitioner before use.

Start with a very small dose, such as one granule of pollen, and build up the dose each day if there are no negative side effects.

Propolis may lower blood pressure in some individuals, so those with a consistent low blood pressure should consult a health-care practitioner before use.

Some people take just a few teaspoons a day of bee pollen and notice health benefits, and some take up to eight tablespoons. Propolis is often taken as a preventative or during an illness, such as colds and flu or tonsillitis as a spray or tincture. It is also beneficial for chronic illnesses such as chronic fatigue syndrome and duodenal ulcers, and can be taken every day.

Bee pollen is a whole, nutritionally complete food that is easy to assimilate.

Mind

Pollen contains a range of nutrients and has an immediate effect as a natural booster and energiser. It can be a perfect alternative to caffeinated drinks that may just jangle an already over-exhausted nervous system, confusing the mind's focus and stimulating tired adrenals, which only adds to the exhaustion. Instead pollen nourishes the nervous system and the endocrine system, allowing for a more natural, consistent feeling of supported energy, improving stamina both mentally and physically and increasing resilience.

The high percentage of rutin in pollen helps to strengthen capillaries and blood flow to the brain. This helps not only to nourish the brain, promoting its functioning, but also to prevent strokes. Pollen has been shown to increase brain function such as memory and concentration, too.

In mild depression, pollen helps relieve lack of energy, lifting mood and strengthening the body as a whole, mentally and physically.

In the elderly, bee pollen helps to shake those feelings of inertia that old age can sometimes bring, helping to keep energy strong and vital.

Body

Pollen and propolis are high in antioxidants, polyphenols, flavonoids and phenolic acids protecting our cells, and especially the liver. They also protect the body from free radical damage, helping to counteract the adverse effects of modern living and its environmental stressors such as pollutants and allopathic medicines.

Pollen's gentle and nourishing ways make it the perfect dietary supplement for those convalescing from acute or chronic illness, helping to support the body's vital force. Pollen helps to increase blood haemoglobin, so it is perfect for those who are exhausted and suffering from anaemia.

Bee pollen contains enzymes that help our digestive system, protecting good gut flora and helping the body to utilise all the nutrients from our food. Its anti-inflammatory properties work to support inflamed and irritated digestive tract problems such as colitis. The antimicrobial and antibacterial properties of pollen help not only to protect our digestive system but also act as an immune-system booster, protecting us from infection. Pollen manages acute digestive disturbances such as diarrhoea, and chronic problems such as constipation.

Pollen and propolis protects the immune system from bacterial, viral and fungal infections such as *E. coli*, and candida. For those recovering after surgery or illness, pollen will ensure support and protection of the immune system.

If you suffer from nausea or lack of appetite due to an illness or pregnancy, bee pollen's high nutritional content is a perfect super food during this time. It is also of benefit to children who are picky eaters with poor diets, to ensure they get all the nutrients they need in order to flourish and protect their immune systems.

If your job involves hard labour or is particularly stressful, pollen will nourish and support the whole body, helping to keep you strong.

Research into using bee pollen with allergies has shown that it protects the mast cells (a type of white blood cell) against releasing histamine by 62 per cent, which protects the body from a foreign substance. Buying pollen locally is an effective way of strengthening your immune system against seasonal and local allergies, so try and source your pollen from the local farmer's market and nearby beekeepers.

Chronic alcoholism reduces many of the body's much-needed

nutrients such as protein, vitamins and magnesium, which can cause exhaustion and other illnesses. Bee pollen supplements these nutrients and prevents problems occurring.

Pollen helps to normalise blood cholesterol, helping to increase high density lipoproteins, the 'good' cholesterol, and decrease low density lipoproteins – the 'bad' cholesterol. It is also thought to have the ability to decrease the clumping of blood platelets.

Pollen's high nutritional content helps support women through the menopause. It eases the negative symptoms of hot flushes, aching muscles and bones and an irritated and stressed nervous system.

Pollen and propolis promotes healing, allowing a wound or burn to heal quickly. Pollen's mild analgesic properties help to ease irritation and pain, while its anti-inflammatory abilities help to calm and soothe the skin. Antimicrobial properties help stop any infection.

Beauty and Spirit

Pollen's high nutritive and antioxidant content gives the skin a healthy glow, helping us to age gracefully. The flavonoids, phenolic acids and phytosterols in pollen and propolis not only help with inflammatory skin conditions such eczema and psoriasis, but also to boost the production of collagen.

Propolis has a mild analgesic effect that helps stop pain and itching in irritated skin and soothes inflammation. It is believed to encourage cell regeneration.

Ten Ways with Bee Pollen and Propolis

Heating bee pollen can cause a loss of its nutrient and enzymatic value, so taking pollen directly, which can be bitter, or adding it to cereal, smoothies, salads and dressings is the best way.

1. Breakfast Topping

The nutty flavour of the flax and toasted sunflower seeds, mixed with the bitter-sweet of the goji berries and bee pollen (with an extra spicy kick from the cinnamon) makes a nutritious addition to cereal, porridge and yoghurt.

1 tablespoon of bee pollen
1 tablespoon of flax seeds
1 tablespoon of toasted sunflower seeds
½ tablespoon of goji berries
1 dessertspoon of ground cinnamon
1 dessertspoon of raw cacao nibs

Place everything in an airtight container and mix together well. Use 3–5 teaspoons for adults and 1–2 teaspoons for children as a topping. It should last for 6 months.

2. Anti-ageing Smoothie

1 avocado, stoned
2 cups of nut milk
1 tablespoon of hemp powder
1 dessertspoon of flax seeds
1 dessertspoon of chai seeds
½ dessertspoon of bee pollen

Put all the ingredients in a blender and pulse a few times for an antioxidant-rich smoothie.

3. Pollen Popcorn

This makes a delicious snack for the whole family.

2 cups of air-popped popcorn
1 tablespoon of melted coconut oil
1 teaspoon of freeze-dried goji berries
2 teaspoons of bee pollen

Add the popcorn to a bowl and pour over the melted coconut oil. Sprinkle over the goji berries and bee pollen. Stir and enjoy.

4. Tarragon, Honey and Pollen Salad Dressing

I love this summery, refreshing dressing and add it to salads and lightly steamed asparagus and broccoli.

1 whole lemon, juiced
Zest of half an unwaxed lemon
1 tablespoon of good clear honey (I use thyme honey)
A few sprigs of finely chopped thyme
A few leaves of finely chopped fresh basil or tarragon
Half a cup of olive oil
1 tablespoon of flax oil
A pinch of sea salt
A dash of ground black pepper
Half a tablespoon of bee pollen

Mix all the ingredients together and drizzle over salads, or raw or steamed vegetables.

5. Homemade Nut, Seed and Pollen Granola

Try making your own granola. It will be much healthier and
have less sugar than the shop-bought kinds.

300g of oats
100g of sesame seeds
100g of sunflower seeds
200g of almonds, roughly chopped
150g of hazelnuts, roughly chopped
5 tablespoons of good quality honey
100g of brown rice syrup
2 tablespoons of coconut oil
1 teaspoon of ground cinnamon
1 teaspoon of ground fennel seeds
200g of raisins
2 tablespoons of bee pollen

Add all the ingredients except the raisins and the bee pollen to
a big bowl. Make sure everything is coated and mixed together.
The coconut oil will melt as you blend the other ingredients
together.

Spread the mixture on a baking tray and bake on a low heat
in a preheated oven at 170°C/gas mark 3 for about 45 minutes.
Turn the granola over and flatten it as it bakes to make sure it
toasts all over. Take out of the oven and leave to cool slightly,
then add the raisins and bee pollen, which will melt slightly
into the granola. Store in a large airtight jar and keep for up to
2 months.

6. Pollen Raw Chocolate

Raw chocolate is a fantastic way to get a natural sugary hit. You only need a little to satisfy any cravings.

80g of raw cocoa butter
60g of raw cocoa powder
30g of raw honey
20g of bee pollen
1 teaspoon of freeze-dried cranberry powder
A silicone mould

Prepare a bain-marie (see page 26) and set it over a low heat.

Grate the cocoa butter into the bowl and let it melt. Then add the cocoa powder and stir thoroughly with a balloon whisk until it starts to thicken. Add the honey and pollen. Take off the heat and stir thoroughly.

Add the freeze-dried cranberry powder. Pour the mixture into the mould and leave in the fridge for up to three hours to set.

7. Herbal Mouthwash

Use this as a preventative against cold sores but also to ease sore bleeding gums. Use as a rinse after brushing your teeth in the morning. It will keep for a year.

½ cup of vodka
5ml of calendula tincture
5ml of echinacea tincture
5ml of myrrh tincture
5ml of propolis tincture

Put everything into a clean dry amber bottle.

8. Herbal Healing Balm with Propolis

This is a wonderful balm for cuts and grazes, fungal infections and soothing irritated skin.

330ml of extra-virgin olive oil
25g of dried lavender
25g of dried plantain
25g of comfrey
25g of calendula
75g of beeswax
1 dessertspoon of propolis
8 drops of lavender essential oil

Heat the olive oil gently in a bain-marie (see page 26). Add the herbs and simmer for 3–5 hours allowing the herbs to infuse. Remove from the heat and strain the herbs from the oil.

Return the herb-infused olive oil to the bain-marie on a gentle heat. Stir in the beeswax until it dissolves in the oil. Allow to cool for a few minutes, then add the propolis before it begins to set, and the lavender essential oil, and stir.

Pour into containers for a wonderful homemade healing balm.

9. Calendula and Propolis Salve for Cuts

Calendula and propolis protect the skin from infection and speed healing.

225ml of calendula-infused oil (The Organic Herbal Trading
  Company sells this, as does Neal's Yard Remedies)
75g of beeswax
10ml of propolis liquid extract
15 drops of rosemary essential oil

Place the calendula oil in a bain-marie (see page 26) and heat gently. Add the beeswax and stir until it is melted. Add the propolis immediately after the beeswax has melted and stir. Remove from the heat and add the rosemary essential oil. Pour into your salve containers.

10. Honey, Bee Pollen and White Clay Mask

This mask rehydrates and detoxifies the skin, helping to ease tired, exhausted skin and treat fine lines and a sluggish complexion.

1 tablespoon of good quality set honey
1 dessertspoon of bee pollen
1 dessertspoon of white clay
1 dessertspoon of argan oil

Mix and apply to a clean, dry face with clean, dry fingertips. Leave on for half an hour and rinse off with a cloth and warm water.

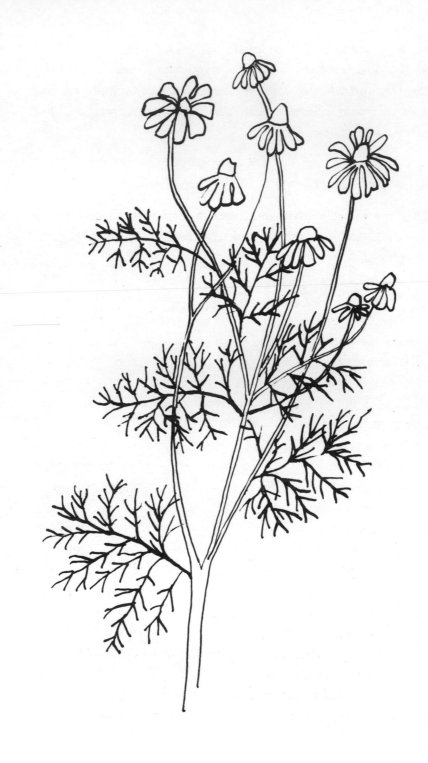

Chamomile

Matricaria chamomilla

Native to: Europe and Asia

My favourite uses: supporting the immune system, digestive and nervous systems, for insomnia, inflammation, anxiety, irritability in children, as a female tonic

You may be wondering why the common chamomile has been added to this book. Chamomile is one of the oldest, most widely used and well-documented medicinal plants in the world. I wanted this gentle yet absolute 'super' herb to have a place here as although it may not have all the incredible qualities of an adaptogen, it does have *all* the right constituents to help reduce the body's reaction to stress by supporting the nervous system and the immune system. This herb can support the whole family emotionally and physically, at every age from baby, toddler, ten-year-old, pregnant mum to the very old, and it is so easy to use in everyday life.

The story of chamomile starts in ancient Egypt, where this small and delicate herb was dedicated to the most powerful and revered god Ra, the god of the sun. The ancient Egyptians believed Ra was swallowed every evening by the goddess Nut, whereupon he would travel through the underworld at night only to be reborn every morning. Thus chamomile was respected as the herb of all herbs that could restore the 'wholeness back to oneself'. The Egyptians would use the herb in their daily life to keep their digestive systems strong and to help allay fever. They'd soak the whole flowers in water as a tonic for beautifying skin and to help prevent ageing.

Chamomile is plentiful in a rich volatile oil and this was used in the embalming oil of the pharaohs, along with frankincense, myrrh, cinnamon, cedar wood, juniper berry and spikenard.

The name chamomile comes from the Greek word *chamaimelon*, meaning 'earth apple', because of its apple-like fragrance. The botanical name *Matricaria* comes from the Latin word for womb because of its healing action for women's health, easing menstrual cramps and anxiety in pregnancy and childbirth (and continuing after the birth to help relax the uterine muscles).

Hippocrates, the Greek physician and founder and father of modern medicine, believed the body should be treated as a whole, not just as a series of parts. He recommended chamomile to treat skin complaints, fever and as a nerve-calming tisane. The scholars of the Classical world – Pliny, Dioscorides, Asclepiades and Galen – all studied and revered this tiny flower.

The Anglo-Saxons used chamomile, known to them as maythen, as one of the nine sacred herbs of the *Lacnunga*, (Remedies), a collection of medical writings and prayers. Chamomile was also used in brewing their staple beverage beer before the use of hops.

'that no one's life be given up to infection, after anyone has prepared him maythen as food' – *Lay of the Nine Healing Herbs*

In the Middle Ages chamomile became a medicinal herb with many uses and was widely cultivated in herb gardens. It was used for respiratory problems, colic and fever, inflammation, skin diseases, digestive problems such as nausea and diarrhoea, and nervous system maladies. It was also used as a 'strewing herb', scattered on floors to add a pleasant fragrance to the home, while acting as an insecticide.

In the sixteenth and seventeenth centuries, physicians used chamomile to relieve many maladies: to stimulate a sluggish liver, ease cardiac diseases, as an antibacterial and anti-inflammatory, a carminative or aid to digestion, and as a healing sedative. It was cultivated across Germany, Russia, France and Hungary, and today chamomile is largely imported from Eastern European countries and Egypt.

Traditionally chamomile has been used to treat an array of ailments, from wounds and viral infections of the skin such as chicken pox to bacterial infections. It was used as a mild sedative for hysteria, sleep problems and anxiety, and as a digestive for diarrhoea, nausea and vomiting. It has been used in the area of women's health to ease painful menstruation and as an emmenagogue promoting menstrual flow, and in treating children with colic, irritability and fever.

Today there are two popular types of medicinal chamomiles commonly used: Roman chamomile, *Chamaemelum nobile*, and German chamomile, *Matricaria recutita*. They belong to different species but are used to treat the same ailments. Easily distinguishable by its daisy-like flowers that bloom between May and October, the German chamomile smells like honey or straw and has longer stems which are singular and upright, whereas its cousin the Roman chamomile smells of fresh apples and grows along the ground with lacy stems, making a wonderful chamomile lawn that is healing to immerse yourself in by walking over it barefoot breathing in the scent.

The chamomile's heady aroma attracts butterflies and bees but keeps most pest insects at bay, which makes them a good companion plant to propagate next to other edible plants to help ensure a good crop. Frances A. Bardswell's *Herb Garden* dubs chamomile the 'plants' Physician'; she wrote that they '*will even revive drooping and sickly plants if placed near them … nature's healer*'. A cold chamomile infusion works well as an organic activator for your compost too.

How Chamomile Can Benefit You

Chamomile is known primarily for soothing ailments of the body's mucous membranes, so it's a perfect remedy for the skin, mouth, throat, gastrointestinal tract and lungs. I look to chamomile for its support with the immune system, the digestive system and the nervous system.

This tiny flower contains many healing bio-active constituents such as terpenoids, flavonoids and, uniquely, azulene, a deep blue, beautiful volatile oil obtained from the flowers by steam distillation, which possesses a whole range of active constituents that play an important role in this flower's anti-inflammatory and healing properties. It also acts as a febrifuge, reducing fever.

Mind

Emotionally chamomile soothes a fraught and stressed-out nervous system. It is incredibly calming and has a mild sedative effect. It's the perfect herb for irritability and fear in children and adults alike, a particularly good remedy for those who have irrational anger and can't quite see further than their own needs and opinions.

Chamomile is also a good herb to take daily for those suffering from anxiety, depression and insomnia. A study conducted in 2009 at the Depression Research Unit in Pennsylvania found that chamomile had positive antidepressant effects on the study's participants.

Added whole or as an oil to a bath it relaxes the whole body, as well as calming a stressed mind and body, helping to induce sleep.

Chamomile also has a calming effect with nervousness in pregnancy.

Body

A chamomile infusion boosts the immune system and helps to fight infections with the herb's antibacterial properties. Inhaling the steam of a chamomile infusion or essential oil in a hot facial works wonders on the mucous membranes of the sinuses when suffering from an infectious cold.

There is a direct link between the gastrointestinal system and the brain, with 90 per cent of our serotonin being produced in our gut lining. Serotonin is a neurotransmitter that helps to regulate our mood, appetite and sleep, and generally contributes to our well-being and happiness. Therefore it is important to have a herb that can help us maintain a healthy digestive system and support any common digestive disorders. A cup of chamomile infusion half an hour before a meal can aid digestion, and after a meal it acts as a carminative to reduce bloating and gas. It's also a perfect remedy for indigestion due to a nervous stomach, and is much better for you and your stomach chemistry for lowering acidity than using commercial antacids.

Chamomile helps relieve nausea, sluggish digestion and diarrhoea, and it's been found to help inhibit *Helicobacter pylori* – the bacteria that can contribute to stomach ulcers. Chamomile helps to reduce muscle spasms associated with various gastrointestinal inflammatory disorders, such as irritable bowel syndrome and colitis. Also, for infants suffering from colic, a warmed infusion of organic chamomile is incredibly beneficial – not just for their tummy but their nervous system too.

There have been many studies of chamomile's anti-cancer effects, and it has been found that the bioflavonoid apigenin, which is found in abundance in chamomile, has potential in protecting the body against cancer. Research with apigenin is being done to induce a process called apoptosis – normal cell death – in some cancer cells. Apigenin also has potential as a cancer chemo-protective agent. It is also a remarkable anti-inflammatory and antioxidant as well as being anti-carcinogenic.

Important note

Please talk to your cancer specialist before taking any herbs and supplements, as they may affect your cancer therapy.

Osteoporosis is a softening of the bones due to hereditary factors, although often poor diet, poor calcium and vitamin D absorption and hormonal changes are also factors. Chamomile has been shown to stimulate and nourish the cells that help build bones, called osteoblastic cells, which is of real benefit to those suffering from osteoporosis.

A study in 2009 confirmed that chamomile's biological make up works in similar ways to non-steroidal, anti-inflammatory drugs helping to prevent inflammation. Studies have also found chamomile to be effective and beneficial in regulating blood sugar imbalances and cholesterol levels.

As a female support, this gentle herb helps relieve the pains of menstrual cramps and helps soothe any tension and irritability during this period; it is also a menstrual regulator. Chamomile is beneficial in soothing pregnancy nerves and sleeplessness, and a safe and beneficial infusion to help with morning sickness and nausea.

Beauty and Spirit

Use topically on skin complaints such as sunburn, irritated rashes, skin eruptions, psoriasis and eczema. It will soothe inflammation and the antiseptic properties of chamomile will help heal the tissues of the skin; anything with heat reacts well to the cooling properties of chamomile. It's also been found to be a wonderful wound healer, helping to speed the healing process of the skin especially in wounds that are slow to heal. A sitz bath of chamomile infusion works well as an anti-inflammatory and astringent for haemorrhoids, and a cooled infusion used as a compress helps inflamed, tired eyes.

Since Egyptian times chamomile has been used in incense as it is thought that burning the herb helps one reach a higher place in meditation and prayer, and in yogic practices to reinvigorate the throat chakra, assisting communication and self-expression. This chakra is also associated with supporting the thyroid and parathyroid glands.

Ten Ways with Chamomile

Important note

Chamomile may cause allergic reactions in those who are allergic to ragweed.

---

1. De-stress Infusion

This infusion will support and nourish the nervous system, helping to ease anxieties from daily pressures.

1 part dried chamomile
1 part dried lemon balm
1 part dried lavender
1 part dried nettle leaves
1 part dried oat tops

Combine all of the herbs in a clean, dry, airtight jar. Take 1 teaspoon per cup of boiling water 3 times a day, or more often if needed. This mixture should keep for a year in an airtight jar.

2. After-dinner Digestif

I rely on this infusion for calming an after-dinner digestive system and for winding down before bed.

1 part dried chamomile
1 part dried meadowsweet
1 part dried spearmint
1 part dried oatstraw

Combine in an airtight container and use 1 teaspoon per cup of boiling water after dinner and or before bed.

3. Salad Dresser

The sweet apple taste of chamomile flowers and their beautiful appearance make them a perfect nutritious topping on a green salad.

2 tablespoons of sunflower seeds
2 tablespoons of sesame seeds
2 tablespoons of chamomile flowers
A pinch of rock salt

Place the sunflower and sesame seeds on a baking tray to roast for 5 minutes at 230°C/gas mark 8. You can also dry toast them in a frying pan on the hob. Let them cool and add them to a jar of dried whole chamomile flowers with a pinch of rock salt. This should last for several weeks in an airtight jar.

4. Chamomile and Astragalus Cough Syrup

This is a delicious way to soothe irritated mucous membranes and relieve a sore throat. Use 1–3 teaspoons every 4 hours when you have a sore irritated chest. The syrup should last for several weeks in the fridge.

50g of chamomile
1 astragalus root (see page 29)
1 litre of water
A pot of good quality honey
1 tablespoon of black cherry compote
A sterilised syrup jar

Place the chamomile and astragalus in a pan with a litre of water over a medium heat and simmer until you have reduced the liquid by half. Strain the herbs and liquid and then pour the infusion into a jug and measure.

Use the same amount of honey as liquid. Place the honey and infused liquid back into the pan and stir on a medium heat for 10 minutes. Remove from the heat and add the black cherry compote.

Cool, bottle, label and store.

5. Chamomile Eye Wash for Tired Eyes

1 tablespoon of dried chamomile
1 tablespoon of dried eyebright

Place the herbs in an airtight jar and make a warm strong infusion by adding 3 teaspoons to a large cup of hot water. Infuse for 15 minutes and then strain, making sure there are no bits of herb left in the infusion. Leave to cool until tepid.

Soak cotton pads in the tepid infusion and place on the eyes for 15 minutes.

6. Headache Roller

I have this simple remedy in my bag for a quick refresher during the day or when I have a strained nervous headache.

15 drops of rosemary essential oil
15 drops of chamomile essential oil
8–10 drops of peppermint essential oil
5ml of vitamin E oil

Combine all the ingredients and place in a roller dispenser (you can buy these online). Roll on forehead and temples when needed, avoiding the eyes. If it does get in your eyes rinse with cold water immediately.

7. Relaxing Bath Soak

This soak is wonderful for irritated skin. I love the honey scent of chamomile and it makes this a truly therapeutic experience.

1 part oats (porridge oats)
1 part oat tops (oatstraw)
1 part dried lavender
1 part dried chamomile whole flowers
10 drops of lavender essential oil (optional)

Mix everything together in an airtight container.

To use, add 1 tablespoon of the mixture to a teapot, fill with boiling water and infuse for 15–25 minutes. Run a bath and then pour the contents of the teapot through a strainer and into the bath, making a bath infusion.

Soak in the herbs for a good half hour.

8. Children's Chamomile Hug (for adults too!)

This gentle mixture is soothing for your baby's (or your) skin.

1 part dried comfrey
1 part dried chamomile
1 part dried lavender

Add a tablespoon of this mixture to a teapot and fill with boiling water. Run a bath for your baby and then pour the strained herbal infusion into the bath, making sure the temperature is perfect for the baby. Allow your baby to soak in the herbs for a good 10 minutes.

9. Chamomile Skin Oil

This soothing oil is a relaxing therapeutic oil to massage on to your skin before bed to benefit the skin and nervous system. The flowers can be fresh or dried, although I prefer fresh.

½ cup of whole chamomile flowers
½ cup of rose petals
500ml of almond oil
20ml of vitamin E oil
15 drops of chamomile essential oil

Mix the flowers and oils and place in an airtight jar. Leave to infuse in a sunny spot for 2 weeks.

10. Hair Rinse for Blondes

This infusion reduces brassiness to enhance golden hair.

2 parts dried chamomile
1 part dried calendula

Add the herb mix to an airtight container and use 1 tablespoon to a pot of boiling water. Infuse for 20 minutes. When tepid pour over washed hair. Leave in – do not rinse off – and dry your hair as normal.

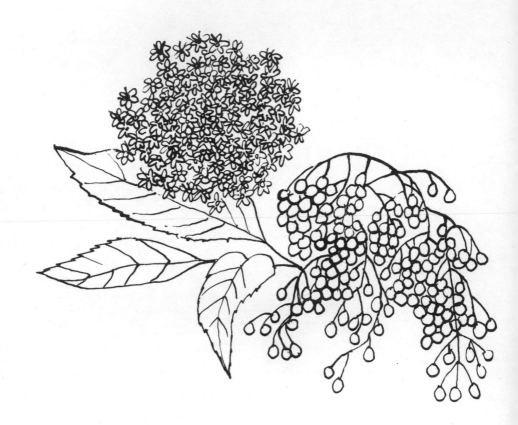

Elderberry and Elderflower

Sambucus nigra

Native to: Europe, North Africa, North America and Southwest Asia

My favourite uses: to reduce fever, as an immune stimulant

I love the name 'elder' as it implies strength and wisdom. Elder is a herb that I use in many of my formulations both for myself and clients – it is a super food and herb with high levels of vitamins A and C and B vitamins, which nourishes and protects the nervous system as well as enhancing and protecting our immunity.

Elder grows wild across Europe, North Africa, North America and parts of southwest Asia in forests, wastelands and damp, wooded areas. It doesn't very much like the heat, preferring swampy, shady places in hotter climes. The leaves, flowers, bark and berries of this small tree or shrub have all been used medicinally for hundreds of years.

You can find elder in parks and open wasteland quite easily. We're fortunate enough to have a mature elder that overhangs our garden that produces beautiful clusters of flat-topped, tiny, cream lace-like flowers that smell fresh and citrusy with a hint of vanilla. They start to appear in my favourite month of May through to July. These blooms are only out for a short period, a month or so, so try harvesting them when the tree is two-thirds covered for optimum medicinal value, and use them medicinally in cordials, wine and infusions and in cooking for their bitter-sweet taste.

Try to pick the flowers in the early morning when they're at their highest potency. Lay them on paper in a warm dry place to dry, allowing any creepy-crawlies that may have been hiding in there to find a new home.

The small green berries appear in the autumn months and turn into dark purple, almost black berries in drooping clusters when ripe, which contain many of the same compounds as the flowers. They shouldn't be eaten when they've not yet ripened – and especially not raw, as they're very bitter and can cause griping, sickness and other gastrointestinal complaints. But when they're dried they're much more palatable, agreeable and medicinal to the digestive system.

The leaves of the elder are dark green with jagged edges, smelling strong and acrid when crushed. They were used as a reliable insect repellant in the past and kept on farms in cow milking pens. Farmers would add a sprig to their hats to keep irritating midges away from their faces.

There's a lot of superstition attached to the elder, most likely because it was supposedly the wood from which the crucifixion cross was made (although the elder is such a small tree I can't see how this could have been true). Elder was used as protection from witches, and the shoots of the elder were buried with the dead to protect them from evil – in fact it was a wood associated with death and the magical. Fairies supposedly celebrate on Midsummer's Eve under it.

It is believed to be a protecting tree and it is good luck to have one growing near your home, especially protecting your back door from evil spirits. A twig of elder kept in the pocket was known as a lucky charm and protection from the pains of rheumatism.

I'm conscious of the superstitions by quietly asking the elder's permission before cutting it back or harvesting the berries and flowers.

A fact about elder that I love that's not medicinal is that the famous Harris Tweed cloth company used the berries for their blue and purple hues, and the yellow from the leaves along with lichen to dye their fabrics.

The berries and flowers are most commonly used today, but historically the bark and the leaves have also been used. The inner bark would be collected in early autumn from the younger trees and used as an emetic. The leaves would be collected in July and used to make a poultice to speed healing. The Native Americans used the elder for infectious conditions, such as viruses, coughs and colds and for healing skin conditions.

How Elder Can Benefit You

The elder has been used in traditional medicine for hundreds of years, and along with rose hips the elderberry has one of the highest antioxidant contents of all the berries – even higher than the well-loved blueberry, cranberry, goji berry and blackberry! Elderberries contain high concentrations of vitamins A and C, and are a rich source of potassium, phosphorus and a good source of iron, assuring the latter's assimilation because of its high vitamin C content. Elderberries also contain tannins, flavonoids, bioflavonoids and triterpenes.

I believe elder has a place among the superherbs and as an adaptogen, helping to increase our natural defences and thereby our overall resistance to illness and stressors. Preparations of elder can be used specifically for an illness, but as an adaptogen the berries and leaves can be used every day to enhance our general well-being and to support the body during periods of exhaustion and excess.

Elderberries have been found to act as a natural immune stimulant and immune modulator, helping to balance the immune system's response. The berries have strong anti-inflammatory and antiviral properties, and are known to be able to halt a virus in its tracks by actually deactivating the enzyme within a virus, stopping it from proliferating within the body.

They are known to be able to do this with ten strains of flu virus.

Mind

Although elder doesn't have a direct effect upon our cognitive health, elderberries' high nutritional and antioxidant value help support overall good health, increasing our resistance when we're faced with stressors. When we feel in tip-top health this has a knock-on effect on how we respond mentally to our surroundings.

Body

The flowers in an infusion make a wonderful diaphoretic for fever, helping the body perspire to eliminate toxins when there's infection, and they are the perfect remedy for fever, colds and sore throats.

In a study it was found that those who took elderberry for flu were seen to recover much faster than those who didn't, and had less severe symptoms; 90 per cent claimed complete recovery after three days.

The berries' deep, rich, dark purple-to-black colour indicates that they are rich in flavonoids including quercetin, and antioxidants – especially anthocyanins that are found in this colour of food. These antioxidants help keep our cells healthy and are especially useful in chronic diseases. Elderberries help to lower the low density lipoprotein, LDL, cholesterol (otherwise known as 'bad' cholesterol) in the blood, helping to prevent atherosclerosis.

Rutin, another flavonoid present in the berries, also plays an important role in our health by helping to strengthen the blood capillaries, therefore strengthening the whole cardiovascular system, improving circulation and preventing vascular disease. An infusion of the flowers makes a good blood purifier when taken daily over several weeks.

The nutritious content of elderberries is believed to help bone formation and they are therefore beneficial for women going through the menopause (and in supporting the elderly).

Elderflowers adapt to our needs. When heated they act as a diaphoretic, helping you to break a fever and sweat out toxins. When taken as a cold infusion, however, they help you to cool down – especially helpful with uncomfortable menopausal flushes.

Post-surgery, both elderflower and elderberry are a wonderful tonic to help boost the body's immunity, enhancing vitality. Elder's antibacterial properties also help protect the body from infection.

Elder seems to have a harmony with the body when treating congestion of the system, whether it be through an allergy, hay fever, infected sinuses or a chest infection. In fact it was the seventeenth-century herbalist John Evelyn who believed elderberry could be used 'against all infirmities what so ever'.

Beauty and Spirit

Historically, the delicate elderflowers have been used in many skin-care preparations because of their gentle toning, soothing and anti-inflammatory properties. They are also believed to give a more even skin tone, helping to prevent fine lines and wrinkles. Elderberries' high antioxidant content also mitigates against the effects of premature ageing, protecting the cell membranes from free radical damage.

Elderflower also acts as a wonderful blood tonic when taken internally, helping to cleanse and detoxify the skin from the inside out. Taken in a cold infusion, elderflower acts as a cooling tonic and diuretic and the berries help to relieve constipation, allowing these pathways of elimination to stay open and for toxins to be expelled by the body. Keeping these channels of elimination open is important for beautiful, healthy skin.

Elderflowers are especially beneficial in healing wounds, burns and skin irritations, and a topical poultice of elderflowers helps to soothe irritated and inflamed skin.

The berries are known to help improve vision in tired eyes, and for sore, itchy, irritated and tired eyes an infusion of elderflowers as a poultice will soothe.

Ten Ways with Elderflower and Elderberry

When harvesting elderflowers, make sure there are no bugs on them by giving them a gentle shake then laying them on paper for a while, allowing anything living there to move on.

When using the flowers take off the green stalks as they taste very bitter and can give you an upset tummy. However, when making a cold infusion it's fine to leave the stalks on. If you want to dry your own elderflowers try not to place them in a bag and leave them as they will not be at their best. Place the clusters face down on clean paper with another sheet on top to protect them from the light.

Taking the berries off their stalks can be very time consuming and fiddly. Try using a fork to pull them off the stem instead, which is much easier and faster.

1. Cold Summer Infusion

Drink this infusion throughout the day for its cooling and diuretic influence on a hot summer's day. It will also help with hay fever symptoms.

Fresh elderflowers
A few fresh mint leaves
Sliced unwaxed lemon

Make a cold infusion by adding a few fresh heads of the flowers to a jug of fresh filtered water or mineral water and leave to infuse for a few hours.

Add a few sprigs of fresh mint and lemon slices if you fancy.

2. Elderflower Cordial

This cordial is delicious, refreshing and high in B vitamins and vitamins A and C. It keeps in the fridge for a few weeks.

1.8kg of sugar
1.5 litres of water
20–30 fresh elderflower florets, with stems cut off
3 lemons, sliced

Put the sugar and water in a pan and bring to the boil until the sugar dissolves.

Place the elderflowers and lemons in a bowl. Pour the hot sugared water over and cover the bowl immediately. Leave for 24 hours to infuse.

Strain the liquid through a wire sieve or muslin and bottle in a sterilised, airtight pouring container. Keep in the fridge and use a small amount at a time, diluting with water to taste.

Try serving with the otherwise discarded lemons or a few mint leaves.

3. Elderflower Fritters

These fritters were a favourite in Elizabethan times and would often be eaten with a sprinkling of fresh sweet cecily, a member of the celery family, with the leaves being used as a sweetener.

Makes 5 fritters

2 eggs, separated
150g of plain flour
½ cup of milk or coconut milk
Vegetable oil for frying
10 elderflower florets

Mix the egg yolks, flour and milk together to make a batter. Leave to settle.

Whisk the egg whites until stiff and then fold these into the batter to make a thick, creamy consistency.

Heat the vegetable oil in a heavy bottomed frying pan and ladle a portion of batter into the oil. Place a floret of elderflower in the batter and fry on both sides till a lovely brown.

Serve with a little sugar and maybe even a little sweet cecily!

4. Elderberry Jam

This isn't just any old jam. It boosts immunity, feeds the body's cells, helps to improve your vision and makes your skin glow!

1 cup of blueberries
1 cup of redcurrants
1 cup of elderberries
½ cup of seedless rose hips, if you have them
1 tablespoon of good quality honey
Powdered cinnamon to taste

Place all the berries and the rose hips in a saucepan. Cover with water to a few centimetres above the fruit. Place a lid on the pan and bring to the boil. Turn down to a simmer until the water evaporates and the berries soften. Remove from the heat and leave to cool.

Depending on how chunky you like your jam, you can purée the berries or leave them as they are, stirring with a fork to mix the berries together.

Mix in the honey and add a little more if it is too tart for your liking. Sprinkle on the cinnamon to taste.

Store in a sterilised jam jar and keep in the fridge for up to 2 weeks. You can also make larger quantities and freeze some or give to family or friends as a gift.

5. Elderflower Wine

This is a classic recipe to make for a May Day. It does need a few months to infuse so keep this in mind!

20 fresh elderflowers, destalked
Zest of 1 lemon

4.5 litres of just-boiled water
1.3kg of sugar
2 lemons, juiced
40g of yeast

Place the destalked elderflowers in a bowl and grate the zest of a lemon over them. Pour over the just-boiled water. Stir, and leave in a safe place for four days.

Strain the liquid using a sieve or muslin. Add the sugar, lemon juice and the yeast. Leave to ferment at room temperature and the liquid will start to bubble from the yeast.

When the bubbling has stopped, stir and allow to sit for another three days.

Strain again through a sieve or muslin and pour the elder-flower wine into sterilised bottles or an airtight container. Leave to sit for three months.

6. Flu and Congestion Relief

I have formulated this blend to treat the common cold, flu, fever and congestion of the lungs and sinuses. It is such a pleasant drink that really helps to eliminate toxins, break a fever, clear nasal congestion and chronic sinusitis, and calm and ease any nervous tension, and upset tummy.

Try to source wildcrafted and organic herbs.

1 part dried nettle leaves (see page 157)
1 part dried elderflowers
1 part dried peppermint
1 part dried cinnamon
1 part dried vervain

Mix all the ingredients together in a bowl and then store in an airtight container.

Use one teaspoon per cup of hot water, or three teaspoons to a pot. Definitely have a hot cup of this infusion before bed to ease a sore throat and to help break a fever.

7. Elderberry Elixir

To keep the immune system healthy try making this delicious elixir. Take 5ml every four hours when you are feeling ill with flu, cough, cold and congested sinuses, or take a teaspoonful every day to help keep you feeling strong and vital.

25g of fresh ginger, chopped (see page 81)
25g of elderberries, dried or fresh
25g of rose hips, dried or fresh (see page 209)
Grated peel of an unwaxed orange
570ml of brandy
A pot of good quality honey

Place the ginger, elderberries, rose hips and orange peel into a large jar and mix well.

Add the brandy until the herbs are covered. Mix the elixir to make sure all the herbs are covered and settled in the jar.

Leave to macerate for 6 weeks. Strain the elixir, discarding all the herbs and mix the liquid with ½ cup honey to each cup of liquid. Leave in a jar for a week to allow the honey to work. Store in an airtight container for 1–2 years.

8. Sore Throat and Mouthwash Rinse

This is a wonderful soothing and antibacterial mouthwash for a sore, inflamed throat or inflamed gums.

3 cups of apple cider vinegar
A handful of sage leaves, washed
4 florets of elderflowers, destalked
2 teaspoons of sea salt

Pour the apple cider vinegar into a clean airtight container and add the sage leaves and elderflowers.

Leave to macerate for 24 hours and strain with a sieve or through muslin. Add the sea salt, place the lid back on the container and shake well.

Take a tablespoonful to gargle and rinse with when you have a sore throat or inflamed gums. This mouthwash should keep for several months.

9. Herpes Salve

Elder has been shown to inhibit the herpes virus, so I have formulated a salve using St John's wort oil to make an effective antiviral, analgesic remedy.

3 tablespoons of sun-infused St John's wort oil
5 fresh florets of elderflower with the stems cut off
50g of natural beeswax
3 drops of lavender essential oil
3 drops of tea tree essential oil

Heat the St John's wort oil in a bain-marie (see page 26) with the fresh elderflowers. Simmer gently for 20 minutes to allow the elderflower to infuse.

Take off the heat and stir in the beeswax until melted. When the mixture has cooled a little, add the essential oils. Before it cools completely and sets, pour the salve into small tins for you to use topically on any herpes sores. This should keep for a year.

10. Problem Skin Tonic

For a clear, even complexion try a daily application of this sooth-ing elderflower toner. It helps remove any excess oils from the skin, removing bacteria and helping to reduce any inflammation. It calms irritated red skin and is perfect for greasy skin that's prone to breakouts. It can also be used effectively in cases of emergency for insect bites, stings and skin rashes. The herbalist Nicholas Culpeper wrote that the 'distilled water of the flowers is much use to clean the skin from sun burning and freckles'.

1 cup of fresh elderflowers
Distilled witch hazel (can be bought from herbal suppliers, see
  page 263 for my favourites)

Place the elderflowers in a jar and fill with witch hazel, making sure the flowers are covered completely. Shake gently for a few seconds.

Store in a cool, dark place for 8 weeks, shaking the jar every day to allow the magical chemical constituents to dissolve from the elderflowers.

Strain the herbs through a mesh strainer after 8 weeks, keep-ing the witch hazel elderflower toner. Squeeze the herbs gently to get every drop of goodness from them, then store the toner in an airtight container and use with a cotton pad when your skin needs it.

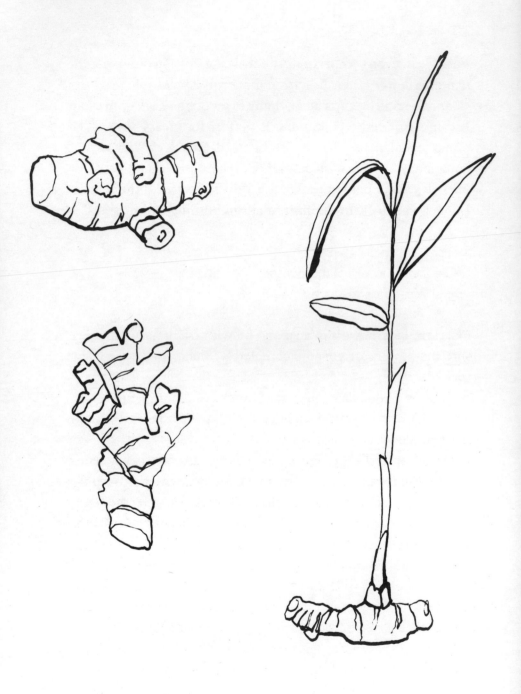

Ginger

Zingiber officinale

Native to: possibly southern Asia and China

My favourite uses: for irritable bowel, as a female/ male tonic, anti-inflammatory, anti-nausea in chemotherapy, loss of appetite

Ginger is world renowned. It is often used in cooking and added to hot water with lemon and honey to treat a common cold. This household spice has an incredible history and has been used for centuries in traditional Chinese medicine and Ayurvedic medicine for so many disorders that respond to its warming strength and decongesting abilities. Also known as the universal herb in Ayurvedic medicine, ancient Indian texts refer to ginger as *mahabheshaj, mahaoushadhi* – 'the great cure, the great medicine'.

Ginger belongs to the Zingiberaceae family, which includes the adaptogen turmeric and also cardamom. The name 'ginger' originates from the Sanskrit word *singaberam*, which translates as 'horn body'. It's not a root, however, but a rhizome, a stem that grows underground. These rhizomes are generally harvested after about six months, but the longer you leave ginger the more intense its flavour. As ginger ages the quantity of essential oils it produces increases. If you use it fresh, then harvest it after five months when it is less pungent. If you are going to use it dried, however, leave it for nine months.

This beautiful, yellow-flowering plant can grow up to 120cm tall. When I was a child my aunt, who did not live in the warm tropical climes of southern Asia but in a draughty cottage in the Lake District, was incredibly proud of growing her ginger plants from the rhizome bought at her local supermarket. She loved saying that never again did she have to pay for ginger as her plant just kept on giving.

No one knows ginger's true origins, but it is thought to be the tropics of southern Asia or from China. As early as 200 BC, ginger's popularity had spread to India, to the spice islands of Maluku in Indonesia, and throughout Asia and West Africa, and it has been used in foods and medicinally by countless civilisations over centuries.

The Romans were believed to be the first to bring ginger to Europe, from their extensive travels through Asia, and they used it to ease their digestive systems after all their excesses. Traditional Chinese medicine practitioners and followers of the Ayurvedic system believed ginger to be a gift from the gods – the use of ginger could enhance spirituality. The Koran describes ginger as one of the heavenly herbs, one of the drinks offered in Paradise: *'and they will be given to drink there a cup mixed with Zanjabil* [ginger]' (Surah 76, v. 17).

These heavenly qualities of ginger may have been one of the reasons, apart from economic ones, that the Arab merchants did not want their ginger trading routes discovered. Ginger was such a lucrative spice that they wanted to protect their trade routes from the Greeks and Romans, who had no idea where ginger came from. They fabricated tall tales of a land called Troglodytia, a fictitious place near the Red Sea which was inhabited by a fierce and deadly tribe of fish-eating troglodytes: ugly cave dwellers. This myth lasted until the thirteenth century when ginger was finally discovered by Marco Polo in China, and by a Franciscan monk called Giovanni da Montecorvino in India.

For thousands of years records show that the ownership of ginger or its trade routes indicated wealth, and ginger has been a trading commodity longer than most spices. Well into the Middle Ages ginger kept its high value, and in England, where its use was known by around the eleventh century, just a pound of ginger was worth the equivalent of a sheep. In Henry VIII's reign ginger was believed to be a preventative and curative of the great plague.

The Spanish took ginger to the West Indies and Mexico to be cultivated and then brought it back to Spain. In 1547 around 22,000 tons of ginger were reported to have been exported back to Spain – this was how important a commodity ginger was!

Ginger was often chosen as an amulet and worn around the neck to protect the wearer from illness and to attract wealth.

How Ginger Can Benefit You

Ginger is an easily accessible adaptogen. Most of you will have this aromatic rhizome in your kitchen or around the corner in your local store, and for this reason I want to extol its incredible virtues here.

Ginger is a delicious, aromatic and fragrant spice. Its warming flavour can be found as a main ingredient in many dishes across the world. It has been used to tenderise meat, and adds a pungent flavour to any dish. It is used in Japan, thinly sliced and pickled, to kill any parasites on raw fish. It is, essentially, a staple spice.

Its unique scent is one that perfume companies have been trying to replicate for years, and its essential oil helps to relieve indigestion, nausea, travel sickness and aching muscles, and to lift spirits. Ginger contains compounds known as 'pungent principles', one being zingerone, and many healing active volatile oils and phenols such as gingerols and shogaols. These have been reported as having an anti-inflammatory, anti-microbial and antioxidant effect and are what helps give ginger its healing kick.

Mind

There have been studies that indicate that ginger root extract may be beneficial in preventing Alzheimer's disease and its debilitating symptoms of memory loss and confusion. There was also an interesting study carried out on middle-aged healthy women that found that ginger extract enhanced their attention and cognitive functions, acting as a gently stimulating brain tonic.

The use of ginger also helps to soothe the nervous system when stressed and anxious, invigorating and strengthening it.

Body

In traditional Chinese medicine ginger is used to expel cold, wind and dampness from the body system and so helps to ignite the body's *qi* or vital energy.

Ginger's most commonly known uses medicinally are to treat digestive issues and colds and flu.

As a hot infusion, grated with a slice of lemon and a good stirring of honey, it is taken for a chill; its antispasmodic properties help a persistent cough. Ginger's diaphoretic action means it has the ability to make you sweat, helping the body release toxins through the skin and (as a mild diuretic) through the urinary system.

Ginger helps to ignite your digestive juices and stimulates the digestive process. It is a popular carminative and stomachic, which means it is an excellent remedy for relieving digestive problems, soothing and settling the gut lining, easing indigestion, flatulence and stomach aches. It is also gentle enough for younger children suffering from colic. It works on the three digestive processes: it helps to increase the production of much-needed digestive enzymes; assists with the absorption of food; and increases elimination. If you have slow digestion try drinking a cup of ginger tea before a meal.

Ginger is a sialagogue herb, which means it increases the production of saliva. It thus helps the start of the whole digestive process, helping to break food down in this first and very important stage which is often missed when we're rushing around, eating on the go, chatting on the phone and so on. This causes no end of digestive disruption which in turn leads to so many other health issues.

Those with chronic digestive inflammatory problems might try ginger to help relieve and calm the symptoms of irritable bowel disease and colitis.

Nutritionally ginger contains vitamin C, amino acids and trace minerals such as calcium, zinc and phosphorus. The herb's synergistic properties also help the body to better absorb these essential nutrients from our other foods too.

Ginger is a well-known remedy used as an anti-emetic, calming nausea and is especially useful for morning sickness. In a trial entitled 'A Controlled Trial on the Open Sea', 80 novice Danish naval cadets were given a gram of ginger each to prevent seasickness. The results were reduced vomiting and reduced cold sweats, and no side effects in contrast to those taking the more commonly used scopolamine. Around 90 per cent of patients receiving chemotherapy suffer from nausea and/or sickness, and there have been many studies over the decades that have proven the benefits of using ginger to lessen the severity and duration of chemotherapy-related nausea.

When travelling, not only does the enzymatic properties of ginger help eliminate parasites – which is something to consider – its antispasmodic properties also help to calm intestinal cramps after an infection.

This stimulating spice helps to improve circulation, and is especially good if you are suffering from chronic cold hands and feet. It can be used on the skin as a rubefacient, drawing a rich blood supply to the skin's surface, helping to get your immune system working by increasing heat to the tissues and bringing relief from inflammatory illnesses such as arthritis and rheumatism. The use of ginger for inflammatory illnesses has been commonplace in Ayurvedic medicine for centuries, and recent studies of inflammatory illnesses of the respiratory system have seen excellent results when treated with ginger.

To keep the reproductive organs firing on all cylinders, take inspiration from ginger, which has been used for centuries as an aphrodisiac. Through the centuries, from China to India and across ancient Greece, people have used the stimulating effects of ginger as a sexual tonic.

Regulating the menstrual cycle and stimulating menstrual flow, ginger is a useful reproductive tonic for both men and women. It directs the flow of blood to the pelvic region, helping to ease any congestion, and its stimulating, analgesic action also helps ease menstrual cramps.

For Malays and Chinese women, ginger is regarded as an essential part of their postpartum recuperation. After giving birth they are encouraged to stay indoors for a month and stay warm with the help of foods containing lots of ginger, such as soups and salted fish with ginger, to stimulate blood circulation and to keep the body warm. This helps the uterus contract to its original size. This thirty-day period is considered vital to a new mum's recovery.

Ginger is used in Ayurvedic medicine to help lower cholesterol levels, and its high antioxidant action is believed to help strengthen the muscles of the heart. Its gentle, stimulating action helps to support the work of the whole circulatory system. Antioxidants, gingerols, paradol and shogaol are key ingredients that can help prevent certain cancers.

Beauty and Spirit

Ginger is a rich source of antioxidants and nutrients that help to protect the skin against free radical damage and collagen breakdown. It also stimulates blood circulation, which is of great benefit for cellulite, and helps to improve elasticity and blood flow, which combats the effects of ageing on the skin. It is also stimulating to the scalp and the hair follicles, helping to stimulate hair growth.

Ginger lifts the spirits and the essential oil is believed to give courage when we are feeling overwhelming fear.

Ten Ways with Ginger

1. Ginger Energy Juice

I love a simple juice, and this one is easy, energising and good for the digestion.

3 organic red apples
2 celery sticks
1 thumb-sized piece of ginger

A handful of parsley
1 teaspoon of Siberian ginseng powder (page 237)

Juice the apples, celery, ginger and parsley. Add the ginseng powder, stir and drink.

2. Ginger, Cloves, Lemon and Cinnamon Infusion

A wonderful way to soothe a cold, enhance immunity, ease stomach cramps and the chills.

7cm piece of whole ginger
1 teaspoon of cloves
1 cinnamon stick
3 slices of fresh unwaxed lemon
Honey to taste

Peel the ginger, grate into a teapot of boiling water and add the rest of the ingredients. Infuse for 15 minutes and then drink. Keep topping up with hot water if needed.

3. Ginger Chicken Broth

This chicken broth can be drunk on its own or used as a base in most soups. As well as the health benefits the ginger adds a little kick.

Serves 2

Vegetable oil for frying
3 shallots, chopped
3 cloves of garlic, crushed
1 carrot, chopped

2 celery sticks, chopped
1 thumb-sized piece of ginger, peeled and chopped
1 tablespoon of peeled and finely chopped fresh turmeric
1 red chilli
4 chicken thighs on the bone with skin
4 bay leaves
½ litre of chicken stock
1 cup of spinach leaves

Pour a few tablespoons of oil into a heavy-bottomed saucepan and cook the shallots until soft.

Then add the crushed garlic, carrot, celery, and spices and stir.

Add the chicken thighs and brown until the skin turns golden. Pour in the chicken stock, cover and leave over a medium heat for half an hour.

Take off the heat, season to taste and add the spinach leaves. Stir and serve.

4. Ginger Syrup

This is sweet and delicious and a wonderful tonic for chills, indigestion, travel sickness and nausea.

50g of ginger root, peeled and chopped
1 litre of water
Honey
1 tablespoon of brandy

Place the ginger in a saucepan with the water over a medium heat.

Simmer until the liquid reduces by half. Strain off the ginger and measure the liquid remaining.

For each ½ litre, add 1 cup of honey. Warm the honey and

the liquid again for 10 minutes. Remove from the heat and add a tablespoon of good quality brandy. Bottle and seal.

Take a few teaspoons when needed. This should last a few months in the fridge.

5. Ginger Gargle

A great way to soothe a sore throat is to grate a 2–3cm piece of ginger and add to a cup of hot water, with a squeeze of fresh lemon juice and ¼ teaspoon of cayenne pepper, whisk briskly with a fork and gargle when the temperature is just right.

You can of course drink the infusion too, but you really want to allow this to do its healing work around the throat first.

6. Women's Relief Decoction

This tea/infusion helps to detox the liver and balance the hormonal system.

1 tablespoon of dried dandelion root
1 tablespoon of dried liquorice root
½ teaspoon of dried ginger root
½ tablespoon of dried chasteberry
½ teaspoon of cinnamon

Mix the ingredients in a sterilised airtight jar.

To make a decoction add 2 teaspoons to a saucepan and heat with 2 cups of filtered water. Add honey to taste, strain and drink.

7. Decoction for Men

To enhance male energy and vitality.

1 tablespoon of cinnamon
1 tablespoon of burdock root
1 tablespoon of Siberian ginseng (page 237)
1 tablespoon of astragalus (page 29)
1 tablespoon of ashwagandha (page 15)
1 teaspoon of black peppercorns
1 teaspoon of ginger

Mix all the ingredients together in a clean airtight container.

Add 1–2 teaspoons to 2 cups of filtered water in a saucepan on the stove and heat for 15–20 minutes. Add honey to taste, strain and drink.

8. Ginger Poultice

To stimulate the stomach, bowels and/or pelvic region, make a poultice of fresh ginger to get heat to this area, igniting its natural fire and vitality.

Simply grate a 7cm piece of fresh ginger and pour over a little hot water to make a paste. Then spread this on to a piece of cotton, fold it over and place it on your belly or pelvis area. Cover the poultice with a cotton towel and place a hot water bottle on top and enjoy the warm, stimulating sensation until it cools.

9. Ginger Body Scrub

This makes a stimulating and uplifting body scrub that's easily prepared in your kitchen. Use sea salt if you don't have Himalayan salt.

500g of Himalayan salt
2 x 2cm pieces of fresh ginger, unpeeled and finely chopped

3 tablespoons of good quality virgin olive oil
A teaspoon of lemon juice

Put everything into your blender and pulse a few times to make sure all the ingredients are mixed well. Then place in a bowl and use in the bathroom, rubbing the mixture on to dry skin with your fingertips or a coarse cloth. Rinse with warm water.

10. Ginger Hair Oil

Ginger's stimulating properties enliven the hair follicles and encourage healthy-looking hair.

Grate a 7cm piece of ginger into a saucepan with 250ml of olive oil. Heat gently, allowing the ginger to infuse with the oil. Remove from the heat and allow to cool.

Strain off the ginger and massage the oil into the scalp. Wrap your hair in a towel and leave the oil on it for half an hour, then rinse and wash your hair as usual.

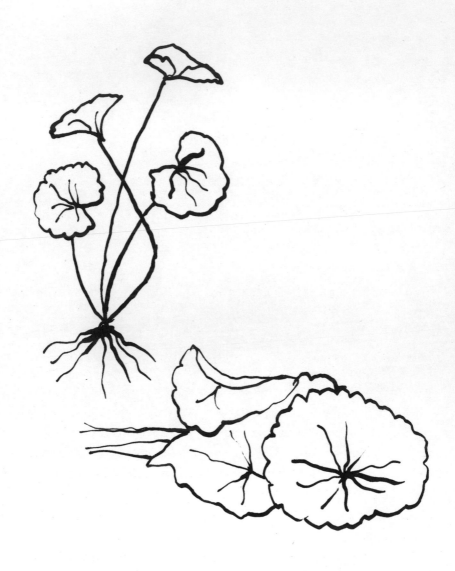

Gotu Kola

Centella asiatica

Native to: India, China and Malaya

My favourite uses: as a detoxifier, relaxant, brain tonic, for wound healing, anxiety

Gotu kola is also commonly called Indian pennywort and belongs to the parsley family, otherwise known as Apiaceae. This creeping herb has small, clustered fan-shaped leaves and these are used medicinally, along with the stems that run along the ground. It is revered in Indian Ayurvedic medicine as having a *'vayasthapana* effect', which means it helps you age with grace and dignity — definitely something to aspire to. It has also been revered for centuries as a *rasayan*: a tonic herb used to strengthen the whole body system.

Gotu kola is believed to have originated in the wetlands of India and in China and Malaya too, where there's a rich history of its use as a herb to improve longevity and vitality; two leaves a day is believed to keep age away.

A Professor and Taoist master, Li Ching-Yun, was a Chinese herbalist reported in official records to have lived to 256, supposedly because of his daily usage of gotu kola. He was reported to have been born in 1677, and to have had 23 wives and 200 children. In 1930 the *New York Times* published an article about him, with documents from Chinese officials congratulating him on his 150th birthday in 1827 and then again on his 200th birthday in 1877. An incredible fable or fact? No one knows, but it does emphasise gotu kola's reputation for helping to sustain a long and fruitful life.

Monks are believed to have used this herb to help quieten the mind to improve meditation, and yogis have historically taken gotu kola to support the brain chakra, balancing the left and right hemispheres of the brain.

Folklore from Sri Lanka tells of the elephant's love of the gotu kola leaves, attributing these leaves to the elephants' famously long lives and astute memories – an elephant never forgets.

Today gotu kola is added to foods in the East in very much the same way as parsley or coriander is added to a Western dish. It can be found throughout Central Asia, China, India, Japan and Sri Lanka, and although it doesn't have a strong flavour or smell, it is known and used as a life-enhancing tonic.

How Gotu Kola Can Benefit You

Triterpenoids are the active constituents in gotu kola. The herb is known for its life-expanding properties, working with the person as a whole improving the vitality of the mind, body and spirit.

It benefits brain function, improves the circulatory system, relaxes the nervous system and improves the body's response to disease and stress.

There have been many studies of the effects of gotu kola on age-related diseases such as hypertension, depression, insomnia, constipation, loss of appetite and cognitive decline, with really favourable improvement recorded.

Mind

There is a belief system called 'the doctrine of signatures' that holds herbs that resemble parts of the body are nature's way of nudging humans in their direction to treat the problems arising in those body parts. It is no coincidence then, that the fan-shaped leaves of the gotu kola plant may be seen as similar in shape to the brain: it's the herb I go to when I see patients who need brain nourishment.

It has been used for centuries within Ayurvedic medicine, from India to traditional Chinese medicine, where it was hailed as 'the fountain of life' and used to improve mental clarity and concentration. For memory loss, nervous stress and a 'chatty' mind and feelings of not being able to think straight (which I myself experience often with four kids ...) to helping with symptoms of dementia, anxiety and mild depression, gotu kola is invaluable.

It has a soothing effect on the nervous system, relaxing the body and especially the brain when it is in overdrive or over-thinking mode, but without a sedative effect. It has also been found to improve brain function and lift mood in the elderly.

Gotu kola has been found to have positive effects with anxiety disorder.

Body

In traditional Chinese medicine gotu kola has been used for a wide range of ailments ranging from infertility to insomnia. It is definitely a herb I'd recommend for its rejuvenating effect on the circulatory system, helping to nourish our whole body system.

It's a powerful blood tonic and detoxifier, and a go-to herb when you have a common cold or respiratory infection. It can be taken daily to help prevent illnesses by keeping the body strong and vital.

For delicate digestive problems, gotu kola has been found to be beneficial in strengthening the digestive mucous lining, reducing the harmful effects of free radicals, and protecting against ulceration.

Gotu kola's ability to improve blood quality and circulation makes it a great remedy for those suffering from varicose veins, working on toning the blood vessels, improving blood flow and reducing swelling. This would also be beneficial for those suffering from chronic venous insufficiency.

A study has suggested that the triterpenoid compound Asiatic acid, derived from gotu kola, inhibits the growth of cancer cells. The triterpenoids in gotu kola also act as anti-inflammatories and have been found to be effective against illnesses such as arthritis.

Beauty and Spirit

Historically, gotu kola has been used to help heal chronic skin problems such as psoriasis, acne and eczema. Its key constituents, triterpenoids, help to heal and strengthen the connective tissues of the body and increase collagen formation. This is especially useful after surgery in helping to speed up healing time, and reducing inflammation and thus helping to prevent scar tissue.

Gotu kola has also been found helpful in preventing and reducing stretch marks and cellulite. Topically it has been found to enhance and speed the healing of burns and wounds without scarring. It is a specific remedy for soothing wounds and ulcers that are slow to heal.

Gotu kola's ability to increase collagen makes it the perfect skin tonic, and the high antioxidant content makes gotu kola anti-ageing too.

Additionally, the herb has been found really helpful for frequent long-haul flyers. Passengers taking gotu kola before a flight experience fewer problems with swollen legs and ankles.

Ten Ways with Gotu Kola

1. Grow Your Own Gotu Kola

This creeping evergreen is easy to grow in our climate. Ask for Duncan Ross of Poyntzfield Herb Nursery in Scotland (see page 263) or look for other reputable specialists in unusual herbs.

2. Green Juice

Try juicing the leaves to promote healthy positive ageing and to improve the brain, digestion, liver and circulation. This recipe might also inspire you to try growing your own gotu kola. If you can't grow your own, add gotu kola to any juice as a powder.

A handful of gotu kola
A handful of watercress
A handful of dandelion leaves
A whole fennel bulb
A thumb-size piece of ginger

Blend all the ingredients together and enjoy!

3. Gotu Kola and Ginkgo Infusion

For an uplifting tea to support cognitive brain function.

1 part dried gotu kola
1 part dried ginkgo
1 part dried rosemary

Mix the herbs in a clean airtight jar, and put 1 teaspoon into a cup of hot water, allowing the herbs to infuse for 10 minutes. Drink twice a day.

4. Nutty Salad Topping

I like to have jars of healthy toppings to hand to add flavour and nourishment to a dish.

1 cup of walnuts
1 cup of hazelnuts
A little coconut oil
1 cup of sesame seeds
1 cup of fennel seeds
½ tablespoon of powdered gotu kola
½ tablespoon of powdered ginkgo
½ tablespoon of garlic powder

Crush the nuts quickly with a pestle and mortar.

Heat the coconut oil in a frying pan, add the seeds and nuts and lightly toast them. Add the powdered herbs and stir.

Take off the heat, allow to cool and store in an airtight container for up to 5 days.

This is also really delicious added to a simple pasta and olive oil dish, or as a topping on potatoes.

5. Sri Lankan Salad

This is a well-known dish in Sri Lanka called gotu kola *sambol* or salad. My husband, Charlie, loves this refreshing and revitalising dish from his travels there.

1 bunch of gotu kola, chopped
5 shallots, chopped
4 green chillies, finely chopped
2 tablespoons of freshly grated coconut (or rehydrate dried shredded
   coconut in water for half an hour)
Juice of half a lime
Freshly ground black pepper
Salt to taste

Wash the gotu kola leaves and place in a bowl. Add the shallots, green chillies and the coconut (or strain the rehydrated coconut and add). Pour over the lime juice, and add salt and pepper to taste. Enjoy immediately.

6. Brain Treats

To keep your mind in tip-top condition and your energy balanced and vital, try these energy balls.

1 jar of nut butter – I like cashew or almond
1.5 cups of honey
40g of gotu kola powder
40g of ashwagandha powder (page 15)
40g of super greens powder
1 cup of cocoa nibs
½ cup of raw maca powder
½ cup of bee pollen (page 39)
1 cup of shredded coconut

Mix the nut butter and honey together in a bowl. Add the goti kola, ashwagandha and super greens powder and stir. Add the cocoa nibs and maca powder and stir again. Use clean palms to roll the mixture into 4cm diameter balls.

Combine the bee pollen and coconut in a bowl and gently roll the balls in the coconut mixture to evenly coat. Place on a baking tray lined with greaseproof paper and put in the fridge to harden (make sure the tray fits in the fridge). Store in an airtight container in the fridge for up to 6 weeks.

7. Gotu Kola and Rosemary Vinegar

Add this vinegar to salads and other dishes as a brain nourishment. This should last in a sterilised jar for up to three months.

A handful of gotu kola leaves
A good sprig of rosemary
A litre of good quality apple cider vinegar

Place the clean dry herbs in the bottom of a sterilised 1-litre Kilner clip-top vinegar bottle and pour the vinegar over them to the top of the bottle. Seal and leave to infuse for up to 6 weeks.

8. Varicose Vein Infusion

Gotu kola helps with blood circulation and prevents blood clots in legs. Try this infusion for healthy veins and to prevent thrombosis.

1 part dried hawthorn (page 117)
1 part dried rose hips (page 209)
1 part dried gotu kola

Mix the herbs in an airtight container, then take 1 teaspoon per cup, 3 times a day, in hot water. Infuse for 15 minutes.

9. Gotu Kola Tincture

For improving brain function and memory, especially during stressful times, try a tincture of gotu kola from a reputable source such as Neal's Yard Remedies, or make your own. It must be used consistently every day for at least 4 weeks before you'll start to notice a positive change.

Using dried leaves of gotu kola, place the leaves in a sterilised dry, glass jar, filling it about two-thirds full. Pour over alcohol – I use brandy or vodka – making sure the leaves are completely covered. Put the lid on and store in a cool, dry, dark place for a few weeks. Shake the bottle gently every few days.

After a few weeks, strain the tincture into a bowl using a fine sieve or through muslin, making sure to squeeze out all the liquid from the herb. Pour the tincture into amber bottles and don't forget to label and date the bottles. It should keep for a few years.

As a rule take 5ml twice a day in a little water for adults. Keep away from children.

10. Gotu Kola Mask

Gotu kola's high antioxidant content makes it a perfect skin tonic to cleanse and boost collagen production.

½ tablespoon of gotu kola powder
½ tablespoon of green French clay
Water or distilled witch hazel to mix a paste

Mix the ingredients and apply to a clean, dry face. Leave on for 15 minutes and then wash off using a clean cloth and warm water. Spritz the face afterwards with rose water.

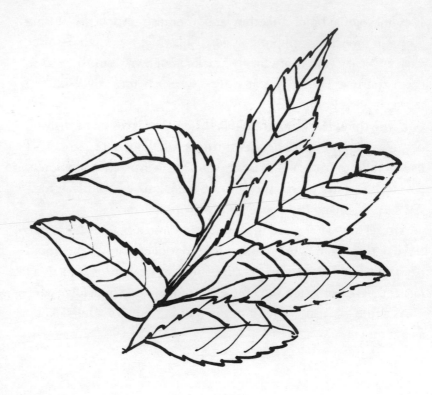

Green Tea and Matcha

Camellia sinensis

Native to: Central and South Asia

My favourite uses: as an everyday antioxidant, for anti-ageing and high cholesterol

Green Tea

Green, black and oolong tea all originate from the same leaves of the *Camellia sinensis* plant. It is the most-consumed drink in the world after water and is cultivated in the southern and central parts of Asia where the temperatures and soil provide the right conditions for growing.

Both green and black tea have been drunk for centuries, with recordings dating as far back as 500 BC in China where it was used primarily as a food, medicinally for treating wounds, in aiding digestion, fever and for calming the mind, and could only be bought in apothecaries.

The custom of tea drinking is believed to have originated

from the mythic Chinese emperor-god Shennong, who devoted his life to seeking the medicinal value of hundreds of plants. A dedicated man, he tried all these himself and is recorded to have reached for tea leaves to cleanse himself of any ill effects.

Something I did not know is that black tea needs some fermentation, when the chlorophyll in the leaves is enzymatically broken down, whereas green tea is produced by steaming the fresh leaves. This stops the oxidation of the leaves and preserves the polyphenols, making it the highest antioxidant tea available. The method of steaming the leaves and buds originated in the eighth century, and later a type of frying was used. Both methods are still in use today to produce the best quality green teas.

Tea drinking was once reserved for the wealthy, and the historic tea ceremonies became part of Chinese and Japanese culture around the tenth century and the Song Dynasty. Tea was so prized it became part of government taxation and special types of tea were produced especially for the royal family, such as Miynlong tea, which would have been presented to the emperor.

By the fourteenth century government taxation of tea was abolished, and by the sixteenth century today's method of dry heating green tea to stop oxidation was introduced. Dutch merchants searching for spices and silk saw the potential of trading this new commodity and started to transport green tea to France, Germany and the rest of Europe in the early seventeenth century, although it was only for the wealthy. From here, our great custom of taking tea that is so ingrained in our English heritage was born.

Matcha

Matcha green tea originated in China and was believed to have been taken to Japan by the Japanese monk Eisai, who encouraged the cultivation of tea trees. He also introduced the Zen Buddhist philosophy to Japan in the twelfth century AD. Green tea drinking and Zen Buddhism have been intertwined ever since and he dedicated his life to cultivating both. Monks would drink matcha to help keep their minds focused, enhancing a calmness in their meditative practice. They also believed, with Eisai, that it promoted longevity.

In Japanese, matcha literally translates as 'powdered tea', and it was Eisai who introduced the way of drinking green tea in this powdered form with a beautiful tea ceremony, and promoted its many health benefits. Matcha grew in popularity and became an aspirational part of Japanese life because of his dedicated efforts. All over Japan appreciation of matcha and its ceremony went alongside art, poetry and *ikebana* – Japanese flower arranging. People at the higher end of Japanese society would employ their own tea masters as an outward display of their wealth and social standing.

The tea ceremony, still famous today in Japan and called *Chanoyu* or *Ocha*, is one of the most beautiful aspects of Japanese culture. The whole ceremony allows the guests a feeling of being honoured, especially the main guest called the *Shokyaku*, in a peaceful, serene environment that has been specially prepared before their arrival. A tea host conducts the ceremony, starting with the cleaning of the ceramics. The tea host's movements can be likened to a form of dance as they go through the ritual of placing three spoonfuls of matcha into each cup and ladling the hot water to make a paste. They then use bamboo to whisk to form the frothy consistency of matcha, which is then offered to each guest in turn.

Eisai believed the tea plants should be sheltered from direct sunlight using bamboo and rice shades and only the best leaves picked for use. This way of cultivating matcha leaves is still used today, with only the supple younger leaves at the top of the plant being picked for use.

The leaves are then air dried and steamed to preserve the vibrant green colour and – more importantly – their medicinal content. When the leaves have dried and are crisp and crumbly they're carefully ground, often by hand so that the leaf temperature can be controlled.

How Green Tea and Matcha Can Benefit You

Green tea has many key health benefits, and matcha is the most potent form of the tea. A good quality matcha tea has between 10 and 15 times more potency in nutrients and antioxidants as regular green tea, but if you prefer a delicious cup of regular green tea then please do continue to enjoy it as you're still reaping the tea's health benefits.

Green tea and matcha are high in polyphenols. These are a large group of plant-based chemical compounds that help maintain your body's wellness. Polyphenols contain at least one phenol grouping, and include phenolic acids, flavonoids and flavonols, to name a few. Many of these polyphenols are known to be high in antioxidants which are known to neutralise free radicals, thereby helping to control the rate at which you age and this helps to prevent a deluge of chronic illnesses such as Alzheimer's and heart disease.

Mind

For centuries green tea has been used for its calming properties; the monks used green tea not only to relax but also to focus the mind in meditation, as it relaxes without causing sleepiness. This is down to its high antioxidant content and to the amino acid L-theanine, which is believed to help with mental stress, anxiety and with physical tension.

A study in 2014 using green tea extract showed positive effects on working memory processing, and the herb may be of use to treat debilitating disorders such as dementia.

Body

The catechins in green tea (another type of polyphenol) help enhance the immune system, together with vitamins A, C and E, zinc, selenium and B vitamins, which all protect the body from viral and bacterial infections.

Regular consumption of green tea may be of great benefit in the prevention of cancer, again thanks to its high polyphenol content. Studies suggest that these polyphenols may act as chemoprotectives. The polyphenols have been found to have the potential to induce apoptosis (programmed cell death) in many types of tumour cells. But, as with all of the adaptogens in this book, please consult your GP or specialist before mixing the herb with other medications.

The polyphenol content of green tea is especially good in protecting the liver from excess, from too much alcohol or from immoderate use of over-the-counter painkillers. As such it is worth drinking regularly if you have to take prescription medications or are undergoing a course of chemotherapy.

The Ohsaki National Health Insurance Cohort Study, conducted in Japan over a period of eleven years and published in the *Journal of the American Medical Association*, involved 40,000 Japanese aged between 40 and 78. The participants who drank more than five cups of green tea daily had a lower risk of dying from a chronic illness, especially of the cardiovascular system, than those who just drank one cup a day; this was particularly positive in women. The polyphenolic content of green tea has been found to be especially protective of the cardiovascular system.

Adding green tea to your daily diet can help in lowering LDL cholesterol, also known as 'bad' cholesterol, and increase HDL high density lipoproteins, the hard-working 'good' cholesterol, helping to prevent atherosclerosis. One researcher, Dr Yoshihiro Kokubo, believes that adding green tea to your daily diet may just make a small but positive contribution to lowering your risk of suffering strokes.

Beauty and spirit

Green tea helps to stop the growth of bacteria in the mouth, helping to prevent tooth decay and bad breath. This doesn't mean you can stop brushing though!

Green tea's high antioxidant content helps to keep the skin looking young and healthy, protecting the skin from environmental pollutants and helping in the prevention of premature ageing and UV sunlight damage.

Green tea and matcha tea ceremonies instil mindfulness and awareness of self, leaving you feeling refreshed and spiritually rejuvenated.

Ten Ways with Green Tea and Matcha

1. Matcha Tea

Although it is now found in most fashionable cafes, not everyone knows how to prepare matcha, so I thought preparation would be a good one to start with.

A ceramic pot of hot water
A cup
Matcha powder (found online or in health-food shops)
Matcha whisk

Heat the water, preferably to 80°C rather than to boiling.

Place a heaped teaspoon of matcha powder in your cup and then whisk the powder with the spoon to evenly distribute the powder. Pour over enough of your hot water to fill the cup three-quarters full, and whisk with the matcha whisk in a W-shaped motion.

2. Coconut Matcha Latte

This quick recipe is a refreshing and rejuvenating beverage. The sweetness of the coconut goes perfectly with the earthy matcha.

1–2 teaspoons of matcha powder
½ cup of boiling water
½ cup of coconut milk
1–2 teaspoons of good quality honey
½ teaspoon of bee pollen (page 39)

Place the matcha powder in a cup (you can sift the powder to ensure there are no lumps). Add a little of the hot water, whisking with a matcha whisk briskly until it is frothy, and then add the rest of the hot water.

Heat the coconut milk gently and add this to the cup while whisking. Add your honey of choice and sprinkle a few grains of bee pollen on the top.

3. Iced Green and Mint Tea

This is a refreshing summer drink to prepare and drink all day to keep you hydrated.

5 teaspoons of green tea
1 litre of hot water

A sprig of mint leaves
A whole lemon, sliced
Ice cubes

Use quality green tea and infuse it with a litre of hot water for 15 minutes, then pour through a strainer into a heatproof jug and leave to cool. When cool add the fresh mint leaves, lemon slices and ice cubes (if you fancy).

4. Green Tea Ice Cream

This was a favourite when I lived in New York, and although this recipe is dairy free and sugar free, it's the real deal.

Serves 2–4

400g can of good quality coconut milk
1 cup of almond milk
1 cup of pitted dates, finely chopped
4 tablespoons of honey
2 tablespoons of matcha powder
A pinch of xanthan gum to thicken

Place all the ingredients in a blender and pulse until the dates have completely mixed with the rest of the ingredients and everything is combined. Leave in the fridge for an hour.

Place the mixture in an airtight freezer container and leave in the freezer for up to 5 hours, opening every hour or so to give it a stir. (Alternatively, use an ice cream maker.)

It will keep in the freezer for up to 4 days.

5. Chia and Green Tea Morning Dish

Not only are chia seeds a great source of omega-3 and antioxidants, they're also high in fibre and a great way to start the day.

2 tablespoons of chia seeds
½ tablespoon of matcha powder
2 cups of almond milk
1 tablespoon of good quality honey
1 cup of blueberries
1 dessertspoon of bee pollen (page 39)

In a bowl place the chia seeds, matcha powder and almond milk, and stir. Leave overnight in the fridge.

The next morning stir in the honey and the blueberries and bee pollen and you have a nutritious, satisfying way to start your day.

6. Matcha Pancakes

Serves 2

100g of buckwheat flour
1 teaspoon of baking powder
1 egg
300ml of almond milk
2–3 teaspoons of matcha powder
Pinch of salt
Butter for frying

Whisk the flour and the baking powder together.

In a separate bowl whisk the egg. Add the almond milk and matcha powder and whisk again.

Add the flour to the egg-and-milk bowl, whisking the whole time. Add a pinch of salt and then heat a little butter in a frying pan and, when hot, pour in a ladle of your pancake mix to make your matcha pancake.

7. Matcha Butter

This is a really tasty spread for your toast. You can also use it on your potatoes or on top of fish or chicken dishes. I like the butter salty but you may prefer to use unsalted.

250g organic salted butter, at room temperature
3 teaspoons of matcha powder

Mix the ingredients together. Mould into a loaf-shape, wrap and place in the fridge to cool.

8. Green Tea and Chamomile Facial Spritz

Use this facial spritz to enliven and refresh your skin during a long day. Rich in antioxidants and soothing, these two herbs make an ideal combination and the fragrance appeals to both men and women.

3 teaspoons of green tea
2 teaspoons of chamomile flowers
1 dessertspoon of distilled witch hazel

Place the green tea and chamomile in a heat resistant bowl with 500ml hot water, and infuse for 15 minutes, then strain and allow to cool. When cold, add the distilled witch hazel and pour into a spritzer bottle.

Label and date, and store in the fridge for a cooling toner.

9. Matcha Face Pack

Matcha's high nutrient and antioxidant content makes this a perfect ingredient for a homemade face pack when the skin's in need of a good cleanse and detox when it's tired and irritated.

1 teaspoon of matcha powder
1 teaspoon of set raw honey

Mix the matcha and honey together to form a paste. Immediately rub on to your clean face and neck using clean fingertips. Wash off after 30 minutes with a clean, warm, damp cloth and enjoy the feeling of vibrant skin.

10. Green Tea and Himalayan Sea Salt Bath

This is a wonderful way to relax and unwind, detox and de-stress. It should keep for up to 4 weeks.

500g of Himalayan sea salt
2 tablespoons of green tea
1 dessertspoon of argan oil
15 drops of sandalwood essential oil

Place the sea salt and green tea in a blender and pulse a few times until mixed. Add the oils and mix, then pour into a wide-mouthed jar. Use a dessertspoonful in each relaxing bath.

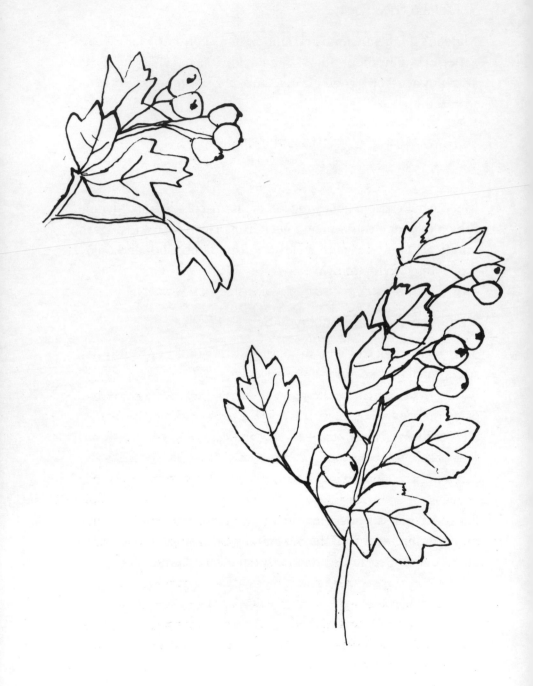

Hawthorn

Crataegus

Native to: Europe, Asia and North America

My favourite uses: as a heart restorative, for anxiety, convalescing, those suffering from a broken heart, unresolved grief

Hawthorn belongs to the Rosaceae or rose family and is the tree of love. It is also known by its Latin name, derived from the Greek meaning 'strength', and is associated with sexuality and fertility.

Another name is May tree and the hawthorn is the only English plant named after the month in which it starts to bloom. Its branches have tough, spiky thorns that are inches long and resemble iron nails that signify protection and caution, and delicate white five-petalled flowers in early spring which have a fetid scent that some liken to the smell of sex! These change to beautiful clusters of small red berries in late summer to autumn.

My dad had a beautiful hawthorn tree over the entrance to his front door, connecting his home to his neighbours'. In fact his road was called Hawthorn Road, although this was the only remaining tree on the street.

In mythology hawthorn trees were thought to be the home of fairies, and according to folklore the hawthorn was believed to have a sacred, protective presence. It was a good thing if a tree stood before a home.

Haw, another word for the fruit, comes from an Old English term for hedge, and hawthorn was used to divide the private lands of England from the common lands. The positive side to the rows of hawthorn that still divide the fields are the many homes they provide for bugs and insects including caterpillars of moths, birds and small mammals, and the fruits and flowers are rich nourishment to them all as well as to humans.

Historically hawthorn was a symbol of fertility, and it was used symbolically in marriage as most ceremonies would take place in May when the flowers were in full bloom. Today it is still seen as sacred and noble because it made up the crown of thorns worn by Christ.

How Hawthorn Can Benefit You

The hawthorn provides nourishment and medicinal properties the whole year round, with its young leaves and blossoms in spring and its berries in the autumn and winter months.

The fruits are rich in vitamins, minerals and bioflavonoids that nourish and protect the heart from free radical damage. Like all adaptogens it can be taken for long periods of time without any toxic effect.

Hawthorn is definitely a herb I use most with my elderly patients to ensure that their cardiovascular system gets the support it needs. I personally use it daily as a tincture and as a fresh infusion in the spring to support and ensure that my heart stays young and vital too.

Mind

Hawthorn treats stress and anxiety by having a mild sedative effect on the nervous system, and by nourishing and regulating the cardiovascular system. It helps to ease the symptoms of anxiety and the 'fight or flight' response. It also helps stress related to heart function such as hypertension, balancing blood pressure and aiding sleep.

Herbs like hawthorn that support the circulatory system improve the cerebral blood flow too, helping with focus and state of mind.

Hawthorn helps the heart stay supported and strong, which in turn gives courage to those anxious in life and those who find it difficult to express their feelings.

Body

After an illness, look to hawthorn to help the whole body recuperate and convalesce, stimulating and nourishing the whole body system – a perfect adaptogen tonic.

In traditional Chinese medicine hawthorn stimulates the spleen, increasing the body's immunity and its ability to purify the blood.

Hawthorn is high in flavonoids – powerful antioxidants with anti-inflammatory and immune-supporting compounds – as well as oligomeric proanthocyanidins (OPCs), a group of flavonoids found in most fruits and vegetables but in high concentrations in hawthorn leaves, flowers and berries. These compounds protect the heart, making hawthorn an incredible heart and circulatory tonic with the ability to adapt the heart's function by gently stimulating or depressing its activity.

As well as being restorative to the heart, hawthorn helps to heal and support the blood vessels and coronary arteries, helping to improve blood circulation around the body, working also on the structure and benefitting those with varicose veins.

As a digestive hawthorn is thought to increase fat digestion and help increase the production of the stomach's digestive enzymes.

Beauty and Spirit

In traditional Chinese medicine, hawthorn has been used for centuries to calm the spirit. *Shen* is the word for 'spirit' or 'mind' in Chinese medicine and when the *shen* is unbalanced it affects our mental and emotional state.

Hawthorn is incredibly healing to the heart in many ways. Those suffering from a broken heart, or who are fearful of loving, will find that hawthorn not only helps to heal the emotions but also allows the heart to open and trust in love and self-love again. It is also a beneficial remedy when there's inner conflict or the feeling of a heavy heart.

The high antioxidant content in hawthorn means it's a useful herb to apply topically to wounds and burns and also to irritated skin conditions such as acne and eczema.

Ten Ways with Hawthorn

Many of the recipes for hawthorn given in this section are to inspire you to go out and forage, connecting you even more to this loving, healing plant all year round.

Important note

Although I have found it safe to use hawthorn in combination with prescription cardiac drugs, I would ask that you seek the advice of your health-care practitioner and herbalist before taking hawthorn.

Children should not take hawthorn.

---

1. Spring Salad of Hawthorn Leaves

The leaves of the hawthorn are some of the first to appear in early spring and are soft and a little nutty when picked. They do get less palatable as they grow older and more exposed to sun, so the emphasis of this salad is the word 'Spring'.

Added to this are young dandelion leaves and wild garlic, which appear around the same few weeks of spring. The blackcurrant leaves, which can be collected all year round, add a fruity, sharp flavour.

A handful of fresh young spring hawthorn leaves
A handful of blackcurrant leaves
A few leaves of wild garlic
A handful of dandelion leaves

For the dressing
1 cup of olive oil
Sea salt or herb salt
Juice of a lemon
A little brown sugar

All the leaves need to be washed, especially the leaves from the ground – dandelion and wild garlic.

Put the washed dried herbs in a large bowl and combine the salad dressing ingredients in another small bowl. Add the dressing to the salad and enjoy a cardio protecting, antioxidant and nutrient-rich accompaniment to any dish.

2. Infusion of Hawthorn Leaves and Blossom

Collect the fresh young leaves of hawthorn when they first appear in spring and the delicate blossoms in May while still white.

Lay your leaves and blossom on clean dry paper to allow any little creatures to crawl out and find a new home, and then leave to dry in a safe dry place on the paper or transfer to a drying tray. They may take up to a week to dry.

When dry, place the leaves and the blossom in an airtight container and take a teaspoonful with hot water during the day.

3. Circulation Infusion

This infusion is a good tonic for the circulatory system, for supporting the heart and improving the mind.

1 cup of dried ginkgo
1 cup of hawthorn leaves and/or blossom

2–3cm of fresh ginger, peeled and thinly sliced (page 81)
1 pinch of cayenne pepper

Put the ginkgo and hawthorn into a clean, dry, airtight jar and give it a shake.

For a warming brew place a few teaspoons of dried herbs into a pot of hot water. Add the sliced ginger and a pinch of cayenne and let it infuse for 15 minutes, then pour yourself a cup.

4. Hawthorn and Cinnamon Liqueur

A lovely immune-boosting, heart-warming snifter to get you through the winter months.

A cup of hawthorn berries (destalked, cleaned and debugged)
1 nutmeg, freshly grated
1 cinnamon stick
Peel of 1 orange (eat the orange; we're using just the peel)
1 cup of honey
500ml of good quality brandy

Put the hawthorn berries, nutmeg, cinnamon, orange peel and honey in a large sterilised jar or bottle, and cover with the brandy, making sure all the ingredients are submerged. Label and date, and leave in a cool dark place for around two years or more – depending if you're patient enough to wait!

5. Hawthorn Apple Cider Chutney

Apple cider vinegar helps with digestion and weight loss, and it lowers blood sugars. If you have dried blossoms it's a lovely touch to add these to your chutney at the end of cooking.

1kg of hawthorn berries (get rid of any mouldy, bruised berries)
½ litre of apple cider vinegar
400g of brown sugar
1 teaspoon of ground nutmeg
1 teaspoon of ground ginger (page 81)
¼ teaspoon of ground cloves
¼ teaspoon of allspice
Clean sterilised jars

Pick the berries from the stalks, wash and drain and place in a saucepan. Pour the apple cider vinegar over the berries and bring to the boil. Reduce the heat to a simmer, cover with a lid and simmer for around an hour.

Remove from the heat and strain the berries. Return the fruit to the pan and add the sugar and the spices and, on a low heat, stir continuously for a few minutes.

Remove from the heat and stir in a few dried hawthorn blossoms if you have them, and place your chutney in clean sterilised jars.

Label and date and enjoy with cheeses and fruit. It should keep for around 3 months stored in a cool place out of direct sunlight.

6. Hawthorn Sauce

A healthy alternative to ketchup but one for the adults only!

3 cups of destalked hawthorn berries
½ cup of apple cider vinegar
½ cup of water
soft brown sugar or honey (as much as you want, to taste)
⅓ cup of black cherry juice concentrate (health-food stores stock
  this; CherryActive is a good brand)

A little sea salt
A pinch of black pepper
A pinch of cayenne pepper (another heart-loving herb)
A sterilised ketchup jar

Place the berries in a saucepan and add the vinegar and water. Bring to the boil, turn down and simmer for 30 minutes. Then turn off the heat and allow to cool.

When cooled, sieve the sauce, removing the skin and seeds of the haws, and return the mixture to the pan.

Add the sugar or honey, to taste. (Some may like it sweeter than others; I would use around one to two tablespoons of honey.) Simmer for another 5 minutes until the sauce thickens a little. Take off the heat and pour in the black cherry concentrate, stirring slowly and continuously. Season with salt and black and cayenne peppers.

Leave to cool, bottle in sterilised jars and store in the fridge. It should last up to 3 months.

7. Foraged Autumnal Jam

A delicious immune-boosting seasonal spread.

Foraged elderberries, rose hips and hawthorn berries
Brown sugar (for 570ml of liquid you will need 450g of sugar)
Juice of 1 lemon
Jam jars, sterilised and warmed in the oven

Haws, rose hips and elderberries all appear around the same time in the autumn months.

Gather around 500g of haws and add about 10 bunches of elderberries and a good few cups of rose hips.

Remove all the stalks from your berries. The easiest way with the elderberries is to use a fork, pulling it down the stalks to make the berries fall off.

Wash all the berries and drain them. Place the berries in a heavy-bottomed saucepan and add 850ml of water. Cover and bring to the boil.

Simmer for an hour and keep stirring and mashing with a potato masher every so often.

When the berries have softened strain the mixture through a sieve or muslin into a bowl.

For every 570ml of juice, measure around 450g of sugar.

Mix the sugar and lemon juice in the heavy-bottomed saucepan and add the sieved berry juice. Bring the mixture to the boil, stirring continuously until the sugar dissolves completely.

Skim off any froth from the top. Remove from the heat and pour into sterilised warm jam jars. Place a cut greaseproof paper circle or a waxed disc on the top of each jar and screw on the lid.

You can eat this jam straight away, no need to wait!

8. Hawthorn Blossom Honey

Herbal honeys are weaker than a tincture but they're still a good gentle medicinal option. And delicious!

You will need a good handful or jarful of fresh dry hawthorn blossom and a jar of good quality clear honey (think 2 tablespoons of blossom to 1 cup of honey), plus an airtight jar.

Collect hawthorn blossoms in early May when they start to appear. Lay your blossoms on a clean sheet of paper, allowing any insects to crawl out and find a new home.

Take a clean, dry airtight jar and lightly pack it with blossom to the top, leaving space for your honey. Then pour your honey over the blossoms, stirring every now and then to make sure all the blossoms are covered and the honey is near the top.

Place the lid on the jar and leave for two weeks in a sunny

spot, tipping the jar back and forth every so often to make sure the honey mixes completely with the blossom.

You can strain the honey and rebottle it after two weeks if you don't want any blossoms. Heat the honey slightly in the jar in a bain-marie (see page 26) to allow for easier pouring.

Don't throw your blossoms away. Leave them in a jar in the fridge for a few days and enjoy sweet hawthorn blossom infusions.

After two weeks you will have your healing hawthorn blossom honey. Enjoy spreading on toast, salad dressings, fruit slices or adding to your infusions or breakfast cereal.

9. A Loving Elixir

An elixir made from hawthorn is guaranteed to promote love!

Hawthorn blossom (fresh or dried, although fresh is best)
A jar of good quality clear honey
A 500ml bottle of good brandy
An airtight clean, dry jar

This is very similar to the Hawthorn Blossom Honey in preparation.

Collect a good jarful of fresh blossom. (Make sure they are collected on a dry day.)

Spread out the blossoms on a clean sheet of paper to allow insects to find a new home, and then fill your jar with them.

Pour in enough honey to completely coat the blossoms. Then pour in the brandy until it reaches the lip of your jar.

Place a lid on your elixir and put it in a dark, cool place for up to 6 weeks. After 6 weeks you can open your jar and strain off the blossom, keeping the liquid and rebottling it. Or you can leave the blossom in – I prefer to keep the herbs in.

Label and date and have a teaspoon of elixir 3 times a day to bring on the love.

10. Healing Hawthorn Tincture

You can tincture the leaf and blossoms in the spring and the berries in the autumn, and then combine them into one tincture for powerful whole-herb healing. If this isn't possible use dried berries, flowers and leaf in one tincture (or, alternatively, make a single tincture of whatever's available to you).

Collect your fresh berries in the autumn or fresh blossom and leaves in the first days of May, giving them a gentle shake and laying them out on clean paper to allow any insects to leave.

Discard any mouldy leaves, berries or blossoms, and destalk the berries.

Place the berries in a sterilised dry glass jar, filling it about two-thirds full. Pour over alcohol (I use brandy or vodka), making sure the berries are completely covered.

Do the same for the leaves and blossom if using these; or use all three, leaves, blossom and berries, if dried.

Place the lid on the jar and store in a cool, dry, dark place for a few weeks. Shake the bottle gently every few days.

After a few weeks, strain the tincture into a bowl using a fine sieve or muslin, making sure to squeeze out all the liquid from the herb. Pour the tincture into amber bottles and don't forget to label and date them. This should keep for a few years.

As a rule take 5ml twice a day, in a little water for adults. Keep away from children.

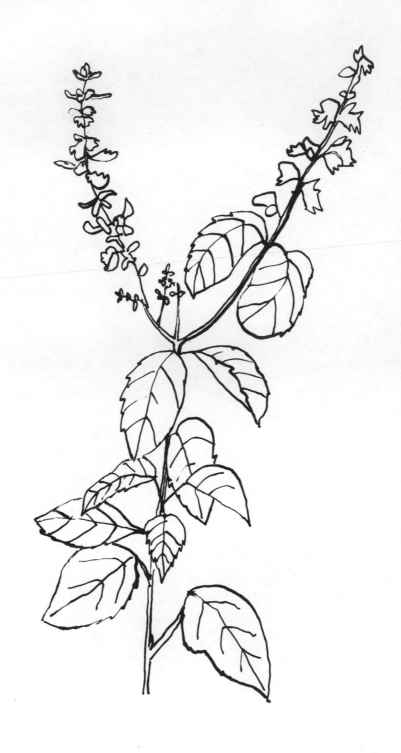

Holy Basil

Ocimum tenuiflorum

Native to: Southern Asia

My favourite uses: as a preventative for all stressors, stopping smoking and use of cannabis, poor digestion, detox against heavy metals, calming a chatty mind

Holy basil, also known as *Tulsi*, the 'Queen of herbs'. Every part of the plant is considered sacred, even the soil in which it sits.

This truly remarkable plant is not only healing and supportive to the body, but is also believed to be nurturing and harmonising to the spirit, giving it the title of 'protector of life'. It is one of the most revered herbs in the whole of India. The leafy shrub is a cousin of the common culinary aromatic basil that we all know and love, and is a member of the mint family.

There are many varieties of holy basil but there are only three that are medicinal. These are 'Rama' – *Ocimum sanctum* – the most commonly used with its purple stems and beautifully green aromatic leaves. This variety has the highest number of medicinal compounds in it, along with 'Krishna' – *Ocimum tenuiflorum* – with its rich purple coloured leaves. 'Vana' – *Ocimum gratissimum* – grows taller than the other varieties and has green leaves and white blossom and a higher percentage of eugenol, which makes it a more effective natural antiseptic than the others. The eugenol content also makes it a perfect indoor plant as it protects the home from mosquitoes and flies.

The sweet-tasting, pungent plant, with its green-to-dark purple leaves that have an aroma of cloves and mint, is found throughout southern Asia and has been revered medicinally for many thousands of years. As the name 'holy' basil suggests, it is cherished as a sacred plant, and its alternative name, 'the incomparable one', reflects how important a herb this is in Hindu culture.

In Hinduism, you'll find holy basil gracing the altars in homes and temples, accompanied with worship every morning to honour the god Vishnu to ensure personal health and family prosperity. It's believed to be the very embodiment of Lakshmi, the goddess of wealth, love and prosperity.

Hundreds of thousands of holy basil plants have been planted around the Taj Mahal to help protect the building from environmental pollutants. This revered seventeenth-century monument is being severely damaged by air pollution from cars and factories, which is turning its famous white marble walls yellow and eroding the marble. Holy basil has been planted in vast quantities to purify and cleanse the environment, minimising the adverse effects of the surrounding pollutants. This gives you some idea of how powerful this delicate-looking plant is.

How Holy Basil Can Benefit You

Holy basil's primary active constituents, eugenol, sesquiterpenes, monoterpenes, vitamins A and C, carotene, calcium, iron, selenium and zinc, balance and nourish the body and its immune system and stimulate anti-inflammatory actions in the body.

In Ayurvedic medicine this delicious sweet herb is a *rasayana*, which means 'path of essence' in Sanskrit. It supports the body on its journey to optimum health. Holy basil works on a deep level, like turmeric, and is believed to be able to shift negative, stagnant energy that inevitably leads to physical and mental ill health.

Where there are fears and stressors in life, unresolved grief and overall disharmony, holy basil acts as a security blanket, supporting and protecting you during these times.

Mind

This spiritual herb has been used in traditional Chinese medicine for thousands of years. It is classified as a *shen* tonic, used to cultivate and nourish mental and spiritual energy. Monks throughout history have been known to drink a warm infusion before long periods of meditation to help quieten their minds of mental chatter and ease the transition into a deep meditative state. The seeds are also made into mala prayer beads, used to help focus the mind in devotional practices.

It helps to calm the mind and is effective for mild depression, insomnia, irritability and overall exhaustion. Used in times of stress and anxiety, holy basil works with the exhausted nervous system. The herb is also believed to have a positive effect on memory and learning, and lifts spirits in the winter months.

Body

Holy basil helps to protect the body from environmental stressors. In Ayurvedic medicine holy basil is recommended to be taken every day as a preventative against disease.

It helps in managing the symptoms of an overstressed body, such as chronic headaches, migraine, tension in the muscles, mild depression, insomnia, irritability and overall exhaustion, by nourishing the nervous system and balancing the endocrine system, improving the body's overall endurance against environmental stress.

An infusion of the leaves has been used for centuries for its immune-stimulating properties and works well in treating all types of infections of the upper respiratory tract and for chronic coughs. It is especially beneficial for chronic chest complaints such as asthma, and infections such as sinusitis, catarrh and ear infections.

High in antioxidants, holy basil has been found to have anti-cancer properties, protecting the body from free radical damage by helping to make these free radicals less toxic to cells. Like most adaptogen herbs, holy basil has been found to protect the body's cells against radiation and chemotherapy damage, enabling a more pronounced positive effect from cancer treatment and a quicker recovery.

Important note

Always speak to your oncologist and herbal specialist before taking any supplements and herbs while on chemo and radiation therapies.

Holy basil protects the body from chemical stress from heavy metals such as lead and mercury, pesticides and industrial chemicals such as parabens and insecticides. It also mitigates against prolonged use of pharmaceuticals such as painkillers and anti-inflammatory drugs.

For stomach cramps, excessive wind and general poor digestion after eating, or even for acute gastrointestinal problems like vomiting, an infusion of holy basil acts as a carminative to soothe and regulate the whole digestive process. It has been found to protect and enhance liver detoxification too, and to help in preventing gastric ulcers, and balancing blood sugars and blood fats.

In Ayurvedic medicine holy basil is used in cases of cannabis and nicotine addiction; its nervous system supporting action helps the stress of drug and nicotine withdrawal.

Holy basil is a powerful yet gentle herb to use where there are a lot of environmental, physical and mental stressors.

Beauty and Spirit

Holy basil has the ability to work on a deep level, balancing all seven body chakras. Chakras (from the Sanskrit word meaning 'wheel') run down the centre of our body from the head to the base of the spine. Our vital energy flows through these chakras, supporting our body's health, rather like the system of meridians in Chinese acupuncture.

A block in the chakras is believed to cause ill health and mental disharmony. Holy basil is thought to help keep energy flowing and aid mental clarity, helping to elevate the spirit and emotions.

Ten Ways with Holy Basil

1. Detox the Home

This beautiful plant is easy to grow and care for from seed and widely available from nurseries and farmers' markets. Its colourful flowers and aromatic leaves need moderate sunlight, and kept indoors it will help combat air pollution within your home.

A sprig can also be dried and burnt to clear the energy in a room at home or in an office space. Or add some to a smudge stick (see page 227).

2. Holy Salad

The leaf makes a nutritious addition to salads. Holy basil has a mild, pleasant taste that doesn't need much added flavour.

1 cup of baby spinach
1 cup of dandelion leaves
1 cup of holy basil leaves
A few calendula (marigold) flowers

For the dressing
1 tablespoon of olive oil
Juice of a lemon
Salt and pepper to season

Wash and dry or spin the salad leaves and calendula flowers. Mix the dressing ingredients and pour over the salad.

3. De-stress Infusion

5 leaves of dried holy basil
1 dessertspoon of dried rosemary
1 tablespoon of gotu kola, dried (page 95)
1 tablespoon of oatstraw, dried (page 169)
1 tablespoon of skullcap, dried

Put all the herbs in an airtight container and mix. Keep for up to three months.

Add 1 teaspoon per cup, or 3 teaspoons per pot, with hot water and drink throughout the day.

4. Cough and Immune-enhancing Infusion

These herbs boost immunity and support the respiratory system and inflamed mucous membranes.

1 tablespoon of dried holy basil
1 tablespoon of dried coltsfoot
1 liquorice stick, chopped
1 tablespoon of dried echinacea
1 tablespoon of dried elderflower

Put the herbs in an airtight jar, stir and seal.

Use 1 teaspoon per cup, up to 5 cups a day, or 3 teaspoons per pot, with hot water and drink throughout the day.

5. Protective Smoothie

I love this easy energy-boosting, liver-cleansing smoothie. This is a revitaliser in the morning or at that 4 p.m. energy dip.

2 cups of nut milk
1 ripe banana
1 teaspoon of dandelion root
1–2 teaspoons of cocoa nibs
½ teaspoon of ashwagandha powder
½ teaspoon of holy basil powder
1 teaspoon of bee pollen

Put all the ingredients into a blender and pulse till smooth. Drink straight away.

6. Holy Basil Water

Add this to a glass with ice and fresh holy basil leaves for a refreshing drink.

½ cup of blueberries
½ cup of raspberries
Juice of 1 whole lemon
Juice of 1 whole lime
1 cup of filtered cold water
½ teaspoon of dried lavender
1 teaspoon of dried rose or fresh rose petals
1 teaspoon of dried holy basil
1 dessertspoon of raw good quality honey

Wash the berries and place all the ingredients in a blender. Pulse until smooth. Pour into a glass with some ice and garnish with a few fresh leaves of holy basil.

7. Courgette and Holy Basil Pasta

This makes a light but filling lunch or dinner dish.

Serves 2

1 cup of small courgettes, sliced
1 medium red onion, finely chopped
3 cloves of garlic, crushed
2 tablespoons of olive oil
250g wheat penne or rice pasta
A cup of ricotta cheese
A handful of fresh holy basil, chopped

Place the courgettes, onion, garlic and olive oil in a small bowl and mix together.

Cook the pasta according to the packet instructions. Take off the heat and drain.

Put the chopped vegetables in a large frying pan and cook until the courgettes are golden and the onions soften. Remove from the heat.

Add the cooked pasta to the frying pan and stir together. Pour the pasta and veggies into individual serving bowls and add a good spoonful of ricotta to each and a sprinkling of holy basil.

8. Thai-inspired Holy Basil Dish

Serves 4

500g jasmine rice
5 cloves of garlic, finely chopped
1 shallot, finely chopped
A large piece of fresh ginger, finely chopped
3 green chillies, finely chopped
1 red chilli, finely chopped
6 shiitake mushrooms, finely chopped
1 handful of fine green beans, finely chopped
1 pepper, deseeded and finely chopped
1 cup of holy basil, finely chopped
Coconut oil, for frying
1 tin of coconut milk
2 fresh limes, juiced
A pinch of Himalayan sea salt
Fresh holy basil leaves to garnish

Place the jasmine rice in a saucepan of water and simmer until cooked.

Heat a little coconut oil in a deep frying pan and quickly fry the vegetables and herbs.

Pour over the coconut milk and the lime juice, and stir over the heat until the coconut milk is simmering. Season with a pinch of salt. Take off the heat and drain the rice.

Serve with a garnish of holy basil on top.

9. Essential Room Spray

A great way to clear the air and energy in a room. These antimicrobial, antibacterial and antiseptic essential oils also lift the spirit and help depression.

10 drops of holy basil essential oil
10 drops of clary sage essential oil
10 drops of lemon essential oil
10 drops of eucalyptus essential oil
20ml of distilled witch hazel

Blend the essential oils in a bowl with the witch hazel and pour into a 150ml amber bottle with a spray. Spray a few squirts around a room to clear stagnant energy when you feel a helping hand is needed.

10. Detox Facial Steam

1 tablespoon of dried lavender
1 tablespoon of dried calendula
1 tablespoon of dried holy basil
½ tablespoon of dried rose petals

Place everything in an airtight jar and shake to blend all the herbs together.

Boil a kettle and add 1 tablespoon of the herbal formula to a heatproof bowl big enough to rest your head comfortably over.

Have a large, clean, dry towel to cover your head and shoulders and then pour the hot water into the bowl with the herbs. Cover with the towel and let the herbs infuse and cool a little.

Then raise the towel and put your head over the bowl with the towel over you.

Close your eyes and allow the cleansing volatile oils in the steam from the herbs do their work. Try to stay there for 5–10 minutes if possible, then come out from under the towel and breathe.

If you fancy repeating this process please do. Then rinse your face with cool water and moisturise.

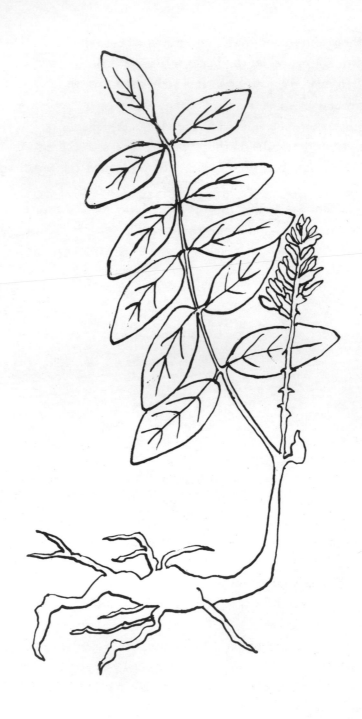

Liquorice

Glycyrrhiza glabra

Native to: Southeast Europe, Asia, China and Russia

My favourite uses: for stress, as a anti-inflammatory, for anxiety with exhausted adrenals, chronic fatigue, inflammatory bowel disease – colitis, chronic cough

Liquorice is a perennial belonging to the pea and bean family. This hardy herbal can withstand many weathers but it prefers the sun and rich sandy soil that are found in its native southeast Europe, Asia, China and Russia. It's hard to find in the UK in the wild, but you may be lucky enough to find it near riverbanks. Look out for its small peapods alongside beautiful spikes of delicate purplish flowers and its graceful oval leaves that look almost feathery on the stalk.

The root is the main part of the herb that is generally used, and these can grow to an astonishing ten metres long and are traditionally unearthed in the late autumn after around four years of growth. The main root that holds up the plant is left and the rhizomes just below the surface are the ones that are cut and used.

Liquorice is also known as 'sweet root' because of its sweet sap, *gan cao* in China and *kanzo* in Japan, and has also been called the universal herb because of its many adaptogen properties – and because it is known and used medicinally throughout the world.

It was considered a superior herb many centuries ago in Britain and during the reign of Edward I in the thirteenth century it was used as a digestive to counter the effects of the fashionably over-rich diet which caused digestive problems and gout. It was in such demand then that a special tax was put on its import. It was first properly cultivated in England by the Dominican friars in the fifteenth century, and cultivated in the Yorkshire Dales where the famous Pontefract cake made of liquorice was manufactured.

This sweet-tasting herb that's not everyone's cup of tea has an interesting history that spans centuries and continents, from China, India, the Mediterranean and North Africa. The ancient Egyptians and their pharaohs used it as a cure-all in a sweet drink called *Mai sus*. Large quantities of liquorice were found among the gold, perfume and precious jewellery in Tutankhamun's tomb to accompany him on the journey to the afterlife.

Chinese liquorice (*Glycyrrhiza uralensis*) has been used since the second century BC and the time of the Han Dynasty. It is known as a primary herb in traditional Chinese medicine and used as a synergist to harmonise and add flavour to other herbs in a formula, as well as to restore and rebalance the whole body system.

In Japan it is one of the most used herbs in Kampo medicine. Kampo is traditional Chinese medicine that has been adapted for Japanese culture over the centuries.

In Greece the herbal physician Dioscorides (c. AD 40–90) gave the root its name, from the Greek *glukos*, meaning 'sweet' and *rhiza*, 'root', and reported in his *De Materia Medica* that the root gave relief from stomach troubles, sore throat and liver and kidney complaints. Nearly 400 years earlier, Alexander the Great's armies reputedly used liquorice root to help alleviate thirst and to give them much-needed stamina on their long, long marches.

Nicholas Culpeper, the famous seventeenth-century herbalist, wrote of liquorice: *'have [for] a dry cough or hoarseness, wheezing and for all the griefs of the breast and lung'*, as it is a wonderful expectorant herb to treat tough chronic coughs and used as an anti-inflammatory on sore, inflamed tissue.

How Liquorice Can Benefit You

Important note

Please note that anyone suffering from hypertension should check with a health-care practitioner before using liquorice, as liquorice in high doses has the ability to induce water retention, which in turn raises blood pressure. I would like to stress though, that this is a gentle herb that children, the elderly and the sick can generally use safely.

Liquorice has a long history of supporting and increasing the body's vitality. It is a balancer and a great harmoniser. I use liquorice in my practice for a variety of ailments from sore throats to constipation, but mainly I find myself prescribing this gem of a herb when there has been long-term 'manageable' stress, causing adrenal weakness over time. This can often lead to feelings of fatigue and exhaustion even after what the patient describes as a good night's sleep.

Sweet-tasting liquorice combines well in a formula, intensifying other herbs' actions and complementing any that have a drying effect or those that have a harsher, bitter action. It has been used for centuries in many traditional Chinese medicine herbal formulas and is known as the 'great adjunct' because of its synergising action.

Mind

I believe a 'mid-life crisis' is not just all in the mind, and should not be taken lightly. Feelings of hopelessness, fatigue, low libido and general uneasiness with life can often be due to adrenal exhaustion after years of pushing the body and burning the candle at both ends.

The adrenals are found just above the kidneys and they produce hormones that affect metabolism, control inflammation, balance the sex hormones, and respond to stressful situations. Liquorice can be a great tonic when they're exhausted – you may be feeling low and foggy.

Body

The active constituents of liquorice contain glycosides that are similar in structure to the natural steroid hormones of the body such as aldosterone and oestrogen. These have a supporting and nourishing effect on the whole endocrine system, especially the adrenals, enabling the body to be balanced and working at its most harmonious.

There has been a lot of research over the last few decades into using liquorice as an antiviral and antibacterial. There's a growing increase in antibiotic resistance, with a real need for us to find alternative ways in which to treat diseases. Liquorice contains triterpenoids, which act as part of the plant's self-defence mechanism, and these are showing much promise as antiviral and anti-cancer agents in humans. Among these compounds are glycyrrhizin (otherwise known as GL) and glycyrrhetinic acid or GA, which have been shown to have inhibiting effects on MRSA, staphylococcus aureus, *E. coli* and candida.

Liquorice has been used for many years in Japan as a treatment for chronic hepatitis B and C and in treating liver disease. Glycyrrhizin is thought to detoxify the liver by helping to improve its filtration of toxins. It has antioxidant and inflammatory properties that protect the liver.

The demulcent properties of liquorice (i.e. soothing effects on the body's tissues) work as an anti-inflammatory, relieving irritating and chronic coughs and catarrh. These properties also soothe irritation of the stomach lining such as gastritis and ulcers.

The polysaccharide constituents in liquorice have an immune-balancing and regulating effect, stimulating where the immune response is lacking and reducing the immune response where there is an auto-immune disease, such as rheumatoid arthritis or allergic reactions.

Liquorice's oestrogenic properties are believed to help some women with uncomfortable menopausal symptoms, primarily hot flushes which can be disruptive to a good night's sleep and reduce self-confidence.

Beauty and Spirit

Liquorice helps to revitalise the adrenals and this in turn restores a person's zest and passion for life.

Ten Ways with Liquorice

1. Natural Toothbrush

Try an alternative to a regular toothbrush and toothpaste and use a liquorice root instead. Its demulcent properties benefit any sore gums or oral ulcers and it is antibacterial as well!

Look for a relatively straight root, not too thick, and chew the end until the outer bark becomes loose and is easily taken off. Continue to chew lightly and soon the fibres will resemble a brush.

Brush your teeth and gums as you would with a normal brush and, if you need to, cut this end off and start the whole process again for the bottom teeth.

Rinse as usual and keep your root in your brush holder for next time.

2. Tasty Spice Rub

I've added liquorice for an extra aniseed taste as a twist on the traditional Chinese Five Spice recipe. Use as a rub for seafood or chicken. This traditional recipe with liquorice and fennel adds an extra digestive benefit.

1 tablespoon of star anise, broken up into smaller bits
1 dessertspoon of fennel seeds
1 teaspoon of crushed cinnamon
1 teaspoon of ground liquorice root
½ teaspoon of ground cloves
½ teaspoon of ground black peppercorns

Blend all the ingredients together and store in a dry, clean airtight container. Label and date. This should last for up to a year.

3. Strengthening Respiratory Infusion

A delicious infusion of antiviral, antibacterial, anti-inflammatory soothing herbs.

1 part marigold flowers
1 part elderflower
1 part coltsfoot
1 part sage
1 part chopped liquorice root

Mix the herbs together and store in a clean airtight jar. This should last for up to a year.

To prepare, place 2 teaspoons in a pot with hot water and steep for 10 minutes. Drink 3–5 cups per day.

4. Dandelion, Burdock and Liquorice for the Morning after the Night Before

For the morning after a night out, have this cleansing liver formula ready on your kitchen shelf.

1 part dried dandelion root
1 part dried burdock root
1 part dried liquorice root
1 part dried sarsaparilla root

Combine the herbs in a clean, airtight container. It should last for about a year.

Make a decoction by adding 3 teaspoons to a cup of mineral or distilled water. Pour into a saucepan, cover and slowly bring to the boil. Then simmer for 15 minutes.

Drink 3 cups a day or until your liver has decided to forgive you!

5. Rehabilitating Tonic

This tonic is perfect after an illness or when you are feeling exhausted. This rich decoction assists the liver, kidneys, nervous and endocrine systems, helping to protect and rebalance them.

1 part dried astragalus (page 29)
1 part dried liquorice root
1 part dried burdock root
1 part dried dandelion root
1 part dried valerian root
1 part dried lemon balm

Put all the herbs in a clean, airtight container and make sure they are mixed together.

Put 2 teaspoons into a saucepan and add a cup of filtered water and simmer for 10–15 minutes to allow the herbs to infuse.

Try a cup 3 times a day.

6. Infusion for the Mature

This is a powerful antioxidant infusion to help increase brain function and vitality in the elderly.

1 part ginkgo
1 part liquorice
1 part astragalus (page 29)
1 part hawthorn flowering tops (page 117)

Put the herbs in a bowl and mix together. Use 3 teaspoons of the mixture to a pot of hot water and allow to steep for 30 minutes. Drink 3 cups daily.

You can keep using the herbs in the pot by adding more hot water.

7. A Woman's Decoction

This formula will help with PMS and pre- and post-menopause and the bewildering symptoms of hormonal imbalance such as bloating, breast tenderness, irritability, poor memory, insomnia, headaches, weight gain and mood swings.

½ tablespoon of chasteberry (found online or in health-food shops)
1 tablespoon of chopped liquorice root
2 teaspoons of a broken cinnamon stick
2 teaspoons of dandelion root
2 teaspoons of fresh parsley (optional)

Put all the herbs in a dry, airtight storage jar and mix. Then put 2 teaspoons in a small saucepan and add a cup and a half of filtered water.

Simmer for 15 minutes, add the parsley (if using) and simmer for another few minutes. Take off the heat and allow the herbs to settle, or strain them using a small sieve. Pour into a cup and start to feel supported.

You can drink up to 3 cups a day, and it may be easier to make enough on the stove for that day and to keep reheating it.

8. A Powerful Cough Syrup

A persistent cough can leave you feeling exhausted. This syrup doesn't just treat the cough, which is often a symptom of an underlying condition, but boosts the immune system too.

25g of liquorice root
25g of fennel seeds
25g of wild cherry bark
25g of echinacea root

25g of marshmallow root
15g of cinnamon bark
1 litre of mineral/filtered water
Around 750ml honey or brown sugar
5 drops of spearmint essential oil
Brandy (optional)

Place all the herbs in a saucepan with a litre of water. Bring to the boil, then turn down to a simmer for 20–30 minutes.

Take off the heat and strain the herbs, preserving the liquid. There should be around 750ml of liquid left.

Add the same amount of honey or brown sugar to the liquid, so 750ml of liquid requires the same quantity of sugar or honey. Place back on a low heat and stir to dissolve the honey or sugar.

Remove from the heat and add 5 drops of spearmint essential oil. You can also add a small quantity of good brandy to preserve the syrup, if you like.

Bottle your syrup in clean, sterilised airtight jars. Label and date.

For adults and children 12 years old and above, take 1 tablespoon of the syrup up to 6 times a day.

Important note

The MHRA, the Medicines and Healthcare Products Regulatory Agency, have advised that echinacea should not be given to children under 12 because of the risk of severe allergic reaction.

---

9. Propolis, Red Sage and Liquorice Throat Spray

A soothing antibacterial, anti-inflammatory throat spray.

You can buy the tinctures from reputable suppliers such as Neal's Yard Remedies. Or you could make a tincture yourself using the method below (see page 25 for more detail on tinctures).

Place one part of each herb in a clean, sterilised wide-mouthed jar until a quarter of the jar is filled with herbs. Pour over the brandy to the very top of the jar, covering the herbs completely.

Leave this to macerate (soften) over 4–6 weeks at room temperature, gently shaking the jar daily to allow the herbs to mix with the alcohol.

Strain the herbs from the liquid using muslin or a fine strainer, preserving the tincture in a new bottle, and label and date, so everyone knows what is in there and when it was made.

An amber bottle is preferable as this helps to preserve the herbs' medicinal properties.

You will have enough here to fill many jars of throat spray and if kept in sterilised airtight containers it should last for 5 years. Be sure to label and date everything.

For a throat spray made with bought, ready-made tinctured herbs, which will make a 50ml bottle of throat spray, use:

3 teaspoons of echinacea tincture
3 teaspoons of liquorice tincture
3 teaspoons of red sage tincture
3 teaspoons of propolis tincture

Mix the above in a clean bowl and use a small funnel to pour into a 50ml spray bottle.

Spray the back of the throat to relieve a painful sore throat 6–8 times a day.

10. Herpes Remedy

Liquorice extract can be used topically to help inhibit the growth and heal the *Herpes simplex*/cold sore virus.

Soak a cotton wool swab in a liquorice tincture and dab the sore several times a day at the first signs of an outbreak.

A good source for tinctures is Neal's Yard Remedies (see page 263).

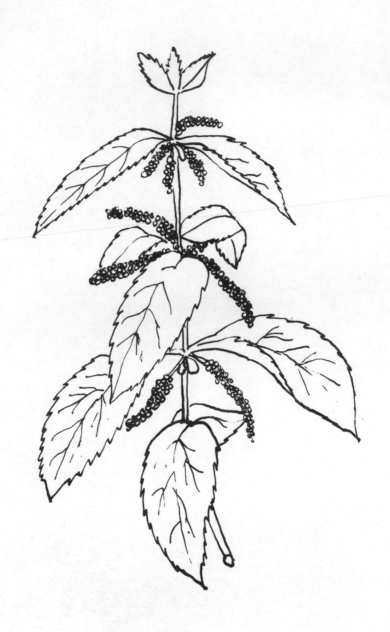

Nettle Leaves and Seeds

Urtica dioica

Native to: Asia, Europe and North America

My favourite uses: for anaemia, allergies, exhaustion, adrenal fatigue, convalescing, cleansing the system, skin, as a diuretic, for breastfeeding, osteoarthritis .

The nettle, or stinging nettle as it is commonly known, is probably one of my all-time favourite herbs. Its Latin name means 'to burn' – more specifically, the burning sensation you feel when you've been stung by brushing against the heart-shaped jagged leaves. This hardy resilient plant, thought of as a weed by many, is actually a nutrient-dense, healing and detoxifying super food, growing all around us on wasteland, in parks and borders for us to easily utilise for healing and nourishment.

From an early age we learn that this herb has a bad reputation; we're told to avoid this plant for fear of being stung. I have to stop myself from shouting warnings to my youngest two when they run along the hedgerows for fear of instilling any negativity about this wonderful herb. There's always a dock leaf nearby to offer relief from its sting, but in the unlikely event one can't be found try rubbing sage or mint leaves on the affected area instead. Even the juice from the nettle itself offers instant relief!

I had help harvesting nettle seeds this autumn from my son Louis. He loved the idea that if ever the situation arose that he was stranded without food, he could live off these nutrient-dense seeds quite happily for a while until he was rescued!

The whole of the nettle plant is beneficial. The tips are at their very best in spring and early summer, but the leaves are not good to use after the nettle starts to flower. The roots should be pulled up when needed in the spring and the seeds harvested in the autumn.

This herb is historically one of the most commonly used herbs in the world. In medieval Europe it was used as a diuretic. Herbalists such as Culpeper used nettle for skin conditions, kidney complaints and gout, and traditionally its juice has been given as a tonic to those debilitated by illness to build up strength and stamina.

Roman soldiers would carry nettles on their long marches as a nutritious food and preventative medicine to allay scurvy, and as far back as the ancient Egyptians, records of nettle have been found in infusions for arthritic pain. Flogging with bunches of nettles, called urtification, was practised to help alleviate the symptoms of arthritic and rheumatic pain – and is still used today by some. Urtification is believed to stimulate blood and heat circulation to the skin, helping to rid the body of toxins. In traditional Chinese medicine, nettle seeds are more commonly used than the leaves and roots for their kidney rejuvenating qualities.

Nettle fibre is similar to flax and has a history of use since the Bronze Age. The strong fibre was used for making sacking, clothing and ropes. During the First World War the German people had to resort to using nettle for clothing fibre when there was a shortage of cotton. Today there's renewed interest in nettle as an ecological alternative to cotton and synthetic fibre. It feels luxurious, like silk, and is not at all prickly.

How Nettle Can Benefit You

Important note

If you are using diuretics or hypotensive medication please consult your GP and herbalist before taking nettle every day.

Many of nettle's medicinal attributes are the result of its dense nutrients, including significant amounts of calcium, iron, magnesium, chromium, potassium, zinc, selenium, silica, manganese, vitamins A and C, B vitamins and high levels of protein. If you're vegan or vegetarian, then nettle is an invaluable addition to your diet to help you stay healthy and vital.

Nettles also contain rutin and quercetin which improves the circulatory system.

Phytonutrients (also known as phytochemicals) within nettle provide us with antioxidants along with flavonoids, helping to enhance our immune response, strengthening our natural resistance. They are also known cancer inhibitors. Look to nettle to basically strengthen and support the whole body system through its cleansing nutritive properties, which enable the skin, kidneys, liver and lungs to work more efficiently in their detoxification processes.

Nettle seeds have been found to be even more nutritious than the leaf, if that's possible!

I use nettle in an infusion every day. Its full green chlorophyll flavour nourishes and cleanses the system and works to support general good health, and the seeds are nutty and delicious sprinkled on cereal. When exhausted they help to give me just the right energy boost.

Mind

Nettle is a superior tonic for treating exhaustion and fatigue. For those who are debilitated by stress and suffering from depression and anxiety nettle's high nutrient and cleansing constituents support the whole body but especially the nervous system. Those finding it hard recovering from an illness and convalescing in need of extra support should look to nettles and nettle seeds to rebalance and re-energise.

Body

Nettle helps to regulate the body's endocrine system, nourishing the thyroid and adrenals and supporting the reproductive system. Nettles make an excellent herb for both men and women wanting to conceive, strengthening the entire reproductive system, balancing, toning and supporting.

When pregnant the herb helps relieve water retention and provides a good organic source of essential nutrients for both mum and baby. If you are breastfeeding and find there's not enough milk being produced, drink a nettle leaf infusion; and if you've too much breast milk it will help reduce this too, so just the right amount of milk is available for your little one.

In menopause nettles help relieve hot flushes, and prevent bone issues in later life such as osteoporosis.

The seeds of the nettle also harmonise the whole endocrine system, but work primarily with the adrenals – especially when you're feeling burnt out and exhausted through stress.

As a blood tonic it is an especially effective remedy if suffering from iron deficiency such anaemia. Nettle is not only rich in iron but also in the other trace minerals and vitamins needed for its proper assimilation.

Nettle supports the body when suffering from allergies such as hay fever and rhinitis, as it has an antihistamine effect. It also helps to calm inflamed, aggravated mucous membranes with its anti-inflammatory properties, helping to eliminate excess phlegm in the lungs where there's a chronic cough, or respiratory weakness and allergies. Nettle also works with other damp, stagnant conditions such as oedema or water retention.

Studies show nettle has had favourable results in reducing high blood sugar, which is of great benefit for those with blood sugar imbalances, and is thought to help reduce sugar cravings by nutritionally increasing energy levels and vitality.

With rheumatic pain, sciatica and weak muscles, try nettle to detoxify, strengthen and nourish. Clinical trials have found nettle of great help to those suffering from osteoarthritis of the hips, knees and hands.

This incredible herb helps as a blood purifier by lowering the level of uric acid in the blood, preventing painful crystal formation in the joints.

For kidney support try using nettle and nettle seeds. In traditional Chinese medicine nettle has been used as a kidney tonic, nourishing, restoring and balancing their yin energy; the leaves have a strong diuretic effect for those who retain water. There has been a positive clinical trial showing that nettle can work as a kidney protective.

There is research into using nettle root in the prevention and restriction of prostate cancer cells, and also positive studies in animals showing that nettle can reduce the toxic effects of the cancer drug cisplatin.

Beauty and Spirit

Nettle's an important remedy when treating chronic skin conditions such as eczema, and is gentle enough for children too. For teenagers with troubling, oily, acne-prone skin, this is the herb to use every day.

Consider nettle as a food for the skin and one of the best herbs in your anti-ageing regime.

With regular use of nettle you'll see stronger and healthier hair and nails as its high mineral content nourishes and strengthens.

Ten Ways with Nettle

1. Fresh Sautéed Nettle Tops

Prepare this in Spring or early Summer when nettle tops are young and tender. This may sound simple but the richness and flavoursome nutty tasting nettle really doesn't need much accompaniment. You can prepare this as a side dish, but I also have this as a main meal as it is so nutrient dense and tasty that it satisfies hunger and the palate.

1 tablespoon of coconut oil
2 cloves of garlic, chopped
4 cups of young nettle tops

Gather your nettles with gloves and wash in cold water, separating the leaves from the stems. Leave them to drain.

In a frying pan heat the coconut oil and cook the chopped garlic cloves. Add the nettle leaves and keep stirring over the heat until the leaves wilt, about a couple of minutes. (I like mine a little crispy.) Remove from the heat and serve with a little salt, pepper and a dash of fresh lemon juice.

2. Raw Nettle and Fruit Juice

Gather young nettle tops. Try to pick from clean environments and wash thoroughly. Blend with other fruits and vegetables (such as those below) for a nutrient-dense juice.

1 cup of nettle leaves
1 apple
½ fennel bulb
2 celery stalks
1 thumb-sized piece of ginger
1 whole unwaxed lemon
1 cup of young spinach leaves

Juice all the ingredients and drink in the morning on an empty stomach to give your liver a treat.

3. Nettle and Spinach Soup

This is a family favourite recipe and is very easy to make.

Serves 4

1 red onion, finely chopped
A spoonful of coconut oil
3 cloves of garlic, chopped
1 large sweet potato, peeled and chopped
1 litre of vegetable stock
A handful of organic spinach
A handful of fresh nettle tops
Salt and pepper to taste
A little grated nutmeg

Put the onion into a heavy-bottomed saucepan with the coconut oil. Add the garlic and fry until both the onion and garlic are soft and a little golden.

Add the sweet potato to the pan, stir for a few minutes, then add the stock and simmer until the sweet potato is soft. Add the spinach leaves and nettle tops and blanch for a minute.

Whizz in a blender, or use a hand blender, until you have a smooth soup. Add salt and pepper to taste with a grating of nutmeg.

4. Nettle and Red Clover Infusion

This infusion is incredibly cleansing and nutritious. One teaspoon helps to allay the effects of allergies and cleanses the blood.

Equal parts of dried nettle and red clover

In order to make a stronger than standard infusion steep a tablespoon of herbs overnight in 500ml of water and strain off the herbs in the morning. Drink throughout the day, heated up on the stove if preferable.

5. Nettle Vinegar

Add this vinegar to salads for a mineral-rich dressing. It should keep in the jar for up to 3 months.

Pick fresh nettle tops (with gloves) in the spring. Make sure you wash them thoroughly and then give them a quick pat dry. Fill a sterilised airtight jar to the brim. Cover with apple cider vinegar and seal.

Leave to infuse for four weeks.

6. Nerve-supporting Infusion

A calming, calcium-rich infusion to support a jangled nervous system. Eases excitability and anxiety and nourishes the body and mind.

1 part dried nettle leaves
1 part dried oat tops/oatstraw
1 part chamomile flowers

Place all the above in an airtight container and use 1 teaspoon per cup with hot water.

Infuse for 15 minutes, drink up to four cups a day.

7. Nettle Seed Harvest

A delicious nutty accompaniment to balance energy when exhausted.

This is perfect in the late summer months when the nettle starts to flower and the leaves are not at their most edible. The flowers slowly begin to ripen into seeds. Wear gloves and start to collect just the green seeds, not the brown ones. It is often easier to pick the whole nettle stem and remove the strands later. Hang these stems or lay them flat to allow the insects to escape, then start to cut off the seed strands.

Lay the seeds flat on a drying sheet for a week in a warm dry place or, even better, use a dehydrator. When dry, rub the seeds through a sieve to remove the husks. You'll be left with the green seeds.

Place these in an airtight jar and store out of direct sunlight, ready to add to soups, juices, cereal and other dishes.

8. Nettle Pesto

Maybe an obvious recipe but I had to mention it here as it is a great, easy way to get nettle into your diet, and sometimes the only way I can get a nutrient-dense dish into my children.

A good bowl full of nettle tops
A good wedge of Pecorino cheese, chopped up
A bottle of cold-pressed rapeseed oil

Using a cloth go through your nettles, taking the leaves off the stalks and then wash well.

Bring a pot of water to the boil and have a bowl of cold water to the side.

Push the nettles into the boiling water for 1 minute, then take out and immediately put them into the cold water. Take them out of the cold water after 1 minute and give them a gentle squeeze. You can do this without gloves as the heat disarms the nettles' sting.

Place the nettles in a blender with the cheese and pulse till blended, trickling in the rapeseed oil as you pulse and get the perfect consistency. Add salt and a little pepper to taste and you have a nutty-flavoured and wholesome meal for the family.

9. Nettle Oil for Problem Hair and Scalp

This powerful infusion is another easy recipe that helps thinning hair and acts as an anti-inflammatory which treats irritated skin conditions, such as dandruff and psoriasis. It is safe to use with sensitive skin.

A cup of chopped nettle leaves
50ml of good quality olive oil

Place the nettles in an amber airtight jar, and then pour over the olive oil to completely cover the nettles. Leave to infuse for a week.

To use, gently rub the nettle oil into a clean dry scalp and massage, making sure you apply it all over the scalp, stimulating blood flow to the hair follicles and skin. Wrap your head in a towel and leave the oil on for a few hours or overnight before shampooing.

10. Stimulating Hair Rinse

This easy to make (although you do have to wait several weeks for the herbs to infuse) nutrient-rich hair rinse stimulates the hair follicles, encouraging hair growth and preventing hair loss. The apple cider vinegar makes the hair healthier looking, smooth and incredibly shiny.

1 cup of fresh or dried nettles
1 cup of fresh rosemary or half a cup of dried rosemary
Apple cider vinegar
10 drops of rosemary essential oil

Put the herbs into a jar with a lid and cover completely with apple cider vinegar. Place the lid on the jar and leave to infuse for up to six weeks in a cool dry place. Pour through a sieve, collecting the herb and keeping the vinegar. Add the drops of rosemary essential oil.

To use, shampoo hair and rinse. Then pour over the vinegar, leave in and dry your hair as usual. Don't worry, when your hair dries there will be no smell of vinegar. (You can also rinse out the vinegar and dry as usual.)

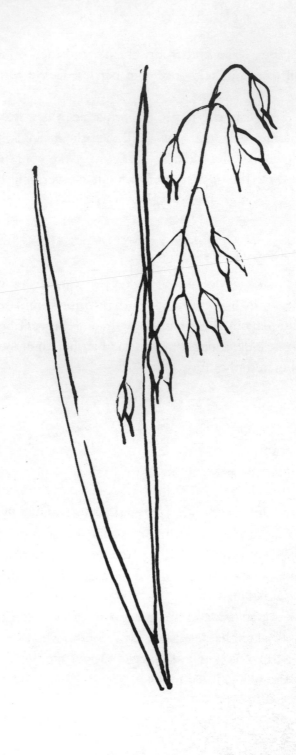

Oat Tops and Stems

Avena sativa

Native to: Europe and Asia

My favourite uses: for exhaustion, anxiety, nervous tension, irritated skin, convalescing

Oat tops are the unripe seed of *Avena sativa*, the cultivated variety of oats. The word *avena* is derived from a Sanskrit word meaning 'foodstuff' and *sativa* comes from the Latin meaning 'cultivated'. Also known as milky oats because of the milky sap that's released when they're squeezed, the tops are picked just after they flower when they're still green. At this time the stalks (or straw) and seeds are medicinal too and can be used along with the tops.

The best time for harvest is just before the grain sets seed when it is richest in avenin – a specific nutrient that works wonders on the cells of the nervous system. This is generally during a one-week period and after this they become the ripe oat that we know so well, which has become a part of our integral food supply, our porridge oats.

Oats prosper in most soils and reach about a metre in height.

They belong to a group of 'panicle forming' grasses, meaning they're not compact like rye and wheat but have loosely grouped grains that catch the light beautifully as they sway and rustle in a summer's breeze.

Oats – or rather the ripe oats – have been a valued part of our diet since prehistoric times. It is believed that our cultivated common oat was developed from the wild oats of Asia, running across to southern Europe. The oldest known wild oat grains were found in Egypt dating from around 2000 BC, and the oldest cultivated source found in Swiss lake dwelling caves dating from the Bronze Age.

Pliny, the Roman naturalist, wrote of the Germanic love for oats, even though his fellow Romans and the Greeks snubbed the common oat, preferring to feed these nutritious grains to their cattle. They believed the oat to be just distorted wheat, although they would use the oats medicinally to bathe sore, irritated skin.

Horses gain their strength from eating a diet of oats and there's much to be said for their nutritive content for humans too. Ripe oats have become a staple in our food history, from Germany across to Scotland, Ireland and England and in the Scandinavian countries. The seeds were taken across to North America with other new crops by Scottish settlers early in the seventeenth century.

How Oats Can Benefit You

Important note

Oat tops are a safe and supportive remedy for everyone, from infants to pregnant and nursing mums to the very sick and the elderly. They may be contraindicated though in those with coeliac disease, so please seek advice from a health-care practitioner before using.

The whole of the oat plant is nutritious as it is rich in alkaloids, saponins, flavonoids, fatty acids and minerals such as magnesium, phosphorus, calcium, folate, manganese, iron, chromium, selenium, vitamins A and C and B vitamins, helping to support the nervous system and keep bones strong and healthy. Of all the grains oats contain one of the highest percentages of protein – up to 17 per cent. There's a unique group of antioxidants that can only be found in whole oats, called avenanthramides. These have a protective effect on the heart, helping to prevent inflammation and high blood pressure.

The tops make the perfect go-to superherb that will support the whole body when feeling totally 'burnt out', exhausted and spent, emotionally and physically. Look to them as a restorative herb to help get the body back on track to feeling balanced and then continuously supported.

This wonderful food for the nerves helps to relax and stimulate the nervous system according to its needs, keeping the body on an even keel in this frantic and stressful modern world, helping us to find our focus, calming anxiety and supporting the cardiovascular system. Think of oat tops as 'food' specifically for your nerves as they have a direct influence on the whole of the nervous system, balancing our vital energy. They act as a nutritive tonic feeding the whole body, but especially the nervous system. I add them to an infusion with chamomile, lavender and lemon balm daily to help keep me supported in this challenging world, and when I'm completely exhausted I know they'll get me back on my feet and back on track physically, mentally and spiritually.

It is the one herb that I have found to work immediately on the body system to calm, support and protect.

Mind

Oat tops' adaptogenic qualities work directly on the nervous system as a gentle stimulant and a mild sedative – they balance and nourish the nervous system's vital force, acting as a restorative and relaxant.

Look to oat tops when the nervous system is completely exhausted and overwhelmed from overwork or from being in a stressed-induced state for too long. Unresolved grief, shock and trauma is enormously stressful, and if not supported can have a negative impact on our general mental and physical well-being. Oat tops help to protect and support a frayed nervous system and endocrine system, allowing space to heal and rebuild our strength and vitality.

In the Middle Ages eating oats was proclaimed a good way to give your brain a boost. Today the use of *Avena sativa* helps cognitive performance. Studies show the positive impacts this herb has on focus, attention and concentration, which may also be considered useful for children with hyperactivity and ADHD.

Oat tops are a good soothing remedy for the relief of tension headaches and occipital migraines due to stress.

Use oat tops when trying to withdraw from nicotine, drug

and alcohol addiction, to help soothe irritability, edginess and anxiety.

Body

The phrase 'to sow one's wild oats' (supposedly first recorded in the 1500s) has always had the sexual connotation of a young man sowing his seed before settling down, but I believe it comes from the knowledge of oat tops' ability to increase sexual libido. They were used in many fertility customs, for example on St Stephen's Day, or Boxing Day, when oats were thrown over young girls with the hope that many seeds would stick to their clothing, reflecting how many children (or lovers!) they would have in later life. Oats were once also used to shower a newly married couple with wishes for their fertile future life together.

Oats help to balance the endocrine system, treating symptoms of PMS such as swollen, tender breasts, feeling exhausted and irritable, insomnia, upset tummy and constipation, headaches, backaches and appetite changes. They also help regulate the menstrual cycle when suffering from amenorrhoea.

These invaluable tops will help calm nervous indigestion and general overall weakness of the digestive system due to stress. They will also help to neutralise excess stomach acidity.

When there's a constant rapid heart rate from anxiety or tachycardia because of stress, oat tops will support, calm and nourish, acting as a cardio tonic.

In the elderly they help support positive ageing by nourishing wasting muscle tone and supporting the nervous system where there are nervous tremors and involuntary body movements, such as with chorea.

Avena sativa's high calcium content supports bone strength, helping to keep osteoporosis at bay and strengthening blood vessels and teeth. Oats also balance blood sugars, supporting those with diabetes and hypoglycemia.

Use oat tops to soothe inflamed mucous membranes, such as with chesty coughs, and to help the digestive system by soothing an irritated stomach and intestines.

Those weak from illness, convalescing or recovering from chemotherapy and radiation therapy, and surgery should incorporate this nourishing herb into their diet. Indeed, whole oats should be thought of as one of the first healing nutrient herbs to help speed the whole body back to strength.

Beauty and Spirit

Oat tops are a perfect remedy for helping to repair the skin after burns and for soothing and calming common itchy skin conditions such as chicken pox, psoriasis, eczema and poison ivy rash. Milky oats are invaluable where there's irritated skin, taken both internally and externally.

As a hydrating bath oats' cooling emollient properties calm an agitated nervous system while rejuvenating and refreshing the skin.

Ten Ways with Oat Tops

1. Juice the Green Oats

A potent 'nerve food' which helps with anxiety, exhaustion and convalescing.

1 carrot
½ cucumber
A handful of spinach

2.5cm of fresh ginger (page 81)
A handful of dried flowering oat tops

Blend or juice all of the ingredients together except the oat tops.
Add the oat tops to a cup of filtered or distilled boiled water.
Strain the water after 15 minutes and add to the juice.

2. Calming Infusion

Oat tops or oat stems are a nourishing addition to a nervine blend. I make the following infusions for my clients.

1 part oat tops
1 part nettle (page 157)
1 part lemon balm
1 part skullcap
½ part lavender

Mix the above in an airtight container and infuse 2 teaspoons per cup of hot water for 10 minutes. Repeat this throughout the day, especially an hour before bed to help the body and (more importantly) the mind to unwind.

3. A Stronger Infusion for Emergencies

Try this strong infusion if utterly exhausted, in shock, or feeling panicked and anxious.
Steep 25g of dried oat tops in 500ml of boiling water for 5 hours or overnight.
In the morning you'll have a nutritious, supporting, nerve-feeding infusion to reheat and drink throughout the day. Just add a little good quality honey to sweeten.

4. Female Supporting Infusion

A nutritional infusion to help keep the hormonal system balanced. High in iron and calcium, this formula is supporting not just during menstruation but every day.

1 part nettle (page 157)
1 part oat tops
1 part red raspberry leaf
1 part dandelion root
1 part liquorice root (page 143)

Mix the herbs together. Use 2 teaspoons per cup and make a decoction on the stove, simmering with water for 15 minutes. Pour into a cup, straining the herbs, and drink up to 3 times daily.

5. A Nutrient Herb Broth Blend

This is a great way to replace shop-bought bouillon for the base of soups and casseroles. It is nutrient dense and these herbs are beneficial to the circulatory, nervous, cardiovascular, reproductive and immune systems.

1 tablespoon of dried oat tops
½ tablespoon of garlic powder
1 tablespoon of dried thyme
1 tablespoon of dried sage
1 tablespoon of dried rosemary (page 223)
1 tablespoon of reishi powder (page 181)
1 tablespoon of marjoram

Put all the ingredients in a blender. Pulse until mixed and add 2 tablespoons to the base of a broth or casserole.

6. Infused Vinegar

A fortifying vinegar; try this to help with the absorption of essential minerals.

½ tablespoon of red clover, fresh or dried
½ tablespoon of nettle, fresh or dried (page 157)
½ tablespoon of oat tops, fresh or dried
500ml apple cider vinegar

Add the herbs to 500ml of apple cider vinegar and leave to infuse.

Add to salad dressings.

7. A Soothing Tincture

Tincturing the oat tops preserves their potency.

Please follow the tincture method on page 25. You could also add other herbs to the tincture, such as ashwagandha to balance and fully support the body, and skullcap for peace of mind.

8. Adrenal Exhaustion Decoction

To increase your energy after a period of exhaustion and to stay supported.

1 part ashwagandha powder (page 15)
1 part oat tops
½ part nettle seeds (page 157)
Honey, to taste

Place the herbs in an airtight jar and then, when needed, add 2 teaspoons to a cup of water in a saucepan. Place on the stove and simmer for 15 minutes.

Add honey to taste.

9. An Emollient Soothing Bath Soak

I like to add oat tops to a bath as hydration relaxation therapy for the body and spirit. The red clay is rich in iron and good for drawing out toxins from the body. It can be found online or in most beauty health shops (see page 263 for my favourite stockists).

1 part oat tops
1 part lavender
1 part rose
1 part chamomile
200g of Himalayan salt
200g of red clay

Mix all of the ingredients together and put in an airtight container.

To use, add 3 tablespoons to a muslin bag, or make a bag by cutting a large square of muslin, placing the herb mixture in the middle and then tying it up.

Leave to infuse in the hot running water and then leave the bag in the bath, squeezing the emollient milkiness into the water for a healing soak.

10. Oat Top Hair Rinse

Oat tops add shine and silky softness to hair. It is also a perfect herb to ease an itchy, irritated scalp.

Infuse 1 tablespoon of oat tops for 20 minutes. Then pour over clean hair as a rinse, massaging into the scalp if needed. Leave the rinse in and dry hair as normal.

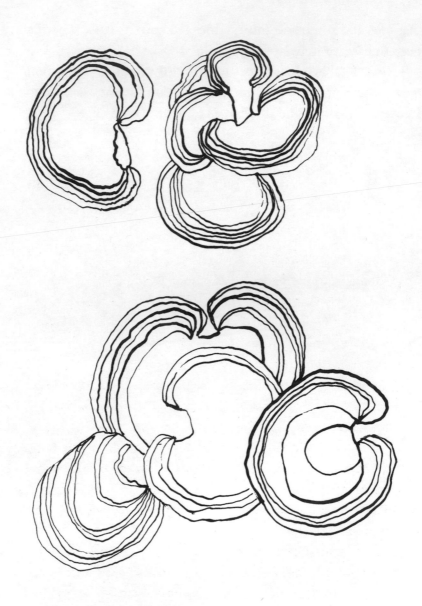

Reishi

Ganoderma lucidum

Native to: China, Japan and North America

My favourite uses: to treat exhaustion, as an antioxidant, for anxiety, cognitive health, convalescing

The name reishi comes from the Japanese interpretation of the Chinese name *ruizhi*, which means 'auspicious mushroom'. Another name from Japan for this mushroom, which I love, is *sarunouchitake* or 'monkey's seat'. Reishi mushrooms have been prized as the 'mushrooms of immortality' for many centuries and they are no doubt the most famous of medicinal mushrooms, especially in the East where they are revered and known as the mushroom of longevity.

Reishi belong to the Ganodermataceae family, otherwise known as shelf fungi, because of their flat appearance. They are woody in texture and brilliantly shiny when wet, almost as though they've had a lick of gloss; their Latin name *lucidum* means 'shining'.

There are various different species within this family, which can be black, purple, yellow and green in colour, but it is the red reishi that are the most researched and therapeutically beneficial. Reishi have small tubes almost like pores, instead of gills, from which they release their spores, their reproductive cells. This is known as a polypore mushroom and can be found, albeit rarely, in the wild at the base of a hardwood tree like maple or oak, elm, beech and birch. But unlike other polypore mushrooms such as chaga, they can survive on both dead and living hardwood.

In the wild there are few high quality reishi mushrooms due to pollution, insect infestation and disease. Probably only 2 or 3 of 10,000 trees have been found to have reishi growing at their base.

Reishi are so rare in the wild that before successful cultivation, only the top nobility could afford them, sending out envoys to find the rare mushrooms in the woods. Due to their rarity, they were immortalised in fine paintings with Taoist healers, carved into wooden furniture and beautifully embroidered on fine silks. They symbolised a successful life and were believed to bring happiness and good fortune – probably because they were often only procured by the rich and privileged.

They have the longest history of medicinal use in China, where they are also referred to as *ling chih* or *ling zhi*, meaning 'the herb of spiritual potency'. These incredible-looking fungi are classed among the most superior of herbs: a source for well-being.

In Li Shizhen's *Bencao Gangmu* (Great Compendium of Herbs) of 1590, considered the first pharmacopoeia in China, reishi was recorded as strengthening the circulatory system, increasing cognitive function, enhancing vitality and generally contributing to a long and healthy life. The Taoist monks who practised traditional Chinese medicine believed reishi to be nourishing to the spirit, a *shen* tonic. They found their use calming to the mind, helping them to focus and concentrate in meditation.

How Reishi Can Benefit You

In Chinese medicine, reishi is a 'spirit plant', the herb that assists in balancing the *jing*, *qi* and *shen* energies: the life-force energy and mental and spiritual health.

Its medicinal uses cover so many of our modern day maladies and chronic ailments, including high cholesterol, high blood pressure, chronic fatigue syndrome, anxiety, leaky gut, diabetes and insomnia. They have been used for centuries to help enhance and extend life, boosting the immune system, and neutralising free radicals that can cause some of these common ailments, preventing premature ageing.

There have been numerous studies of the benefits of reishi since the 1970s, which is when the Japanese started to commercially cultivate this remarkable mushroom. Since then there have been many health benefits found in this adaptogen herb that have justified its traditional use over the centuries.

Mind

Reishi supports the whole body system, helping the mind and body adapt to the everyday stresses of life by supporting the nervous system and replenishing the body's *qi* or vital energy. Reishi eases the mind, helping relieve insomnia, heart palpitations and shortness of breath, which are often symptoms of anxiety, nervousness and over-stimulated adrenal glands.

The high antioxidant constituents of reishi are thought to protect the hippocampus, the part of the brain believed to be the centre of emotion, memory and the autonomic nervous system. It is thought to stimulate cognitive function by increasing blood flow to the brain and acting as a neuroprotector.

Body

Rich in polysaccharides, flavonoids, triterpenes and sterols, reishi is a remarkably beneficial herb for those who are completely exhausted by life – those who have too many stresses to deal with, causing their vital energy to spiral to an all-time low. This can provoke a general feeling of no energy, depletion and a lack of inspiration. Reishi helps prevent the body getting to this point by enhancing the immune system and lifting the whole body system. Working with the immune system is important because if it's found to be overreacting it can often cause chronic health issues, such as allergies and auto-immune diseases. It is often better to try and work with the root cause of the problem rather than just treating the symptoms, and working directly with the immune system helps to rebalance and strengthen the whole body.

Reishi also acts as an 'adjunct therapy', improving overall health when taken alongside other medications for illnesses such as hepatitis and chronic fatigue syndrome. In fact reishi is one of the main ingredients in Fu Zheng therapy, which can be translated to mean 'to restore normalcy and balance to the body'. Some of the other herbs used are astragalus, Asian ginseng, cordyseps, liquorice root and suma root. Fu Zheng doesn't work to fight an infection or disease or its symptoms. Instead, it works directly with the whole body system, strengthening the body's vital energy and its resistance in fighting disease, acting as an immunomodulatory, activating the body's immune response.

Reishi is the subject of many scientific studies of cancer-related therapies, because of the abilities of its constituents (such as beta-glucans and polysaccharides) to not only protect against cancer occurring, but also to stop cancer cells from spreading and metastasising. Researchers at Memorial Sloan Kettering Cancer Center in New York believe that although there is no evidence to support reishi's use as a first-line cancer treatment, they do believe it may have a role in stimulating the body's immune response and therefore have the capacity to enhance treatment. More research is needed to determine its safety and effectiveness in cancer treatment. However the Japanese government officially recognises reishi use within treatments for cancer.

Important note

Always seek the advice of your cancer specialist before taking any herbal therapies and supplements, as they may interfere with your cancer therapy.

Reishi has been used with great success for centuries in the treatment of chronic respiratory illnesses such as allergies and asthma, and more acute problems such as bronchitis, cold and flu. Japanese researchers believe it acts rather like antihistamine because of a compound called lanostan found in reishi, which helps prevent the release of histamine from mast cells within the body, reducing allergic reactions.

The herbalist Lesley Tierra recommends taking reishi combined with astragalus to reduce extreme food sensitivities.

High blood pressure is one of the most common chronic illnesses in our modern world. Reishi can play an important part in supporting our cardiovascular health by improving blood flow, oxygenating the blood (which is useful in extreme conditions such as altitude sickness), helping to lower blood pressure and LDL 'bad' cholesterol levels, lessening the tendency for blood to clot and reducing the risk of heart attacks and strokes.

The high triterpene content found in reishi is also thought to act as a liver protector, helping the body regenerate healthy liver cells. Protecting and supporting the liver and decreasing the level of toxins in our body is incredibly important to our overall health and well-being.

Beauty and Spirit

Reishi contains concentrations of trace minerals and antioxidants which help to oxygenate the cells, nourishing and improving circulation. These benefit many skin problems such as puffiness, dryness, pigmentation, sensitivity and fine lines and wrinkles.

The mushrooms also work hard as antioxidants and detoxifiers against environmental stressors such as heavy metals like mercury and lead.

'They dose themselves with the germ of gold and jade and eat the finest fruits of the purple polypore fungus ... by eating what is germinal their bodies are lightened and they are capable of spiritual transcendence.' (Wang Chong, Chinese philosopher, c. AD 100)

Ten Ways with Reishi

There are lots of ways to prepare Reishi mushrooms. Reishi is really a medicinal mushroom and is not often used in cooking.

It is soft when fresh, but when dried its woody texture is very hard and it tastes very bitter. Many don't mind the taste and use reishi whole or in slices in tea and soups. For those who find the taste too bitter there are lots of capsules, extracts and powders that can be taken instead. It is, however, important when buying reishi to make sure you check it's from a reputable source and, as with all herbs, try to only buy organic.

Wild reishi is believed to have more positive *shen* energy than cultivated varieties. It should be grown and harvested in high altitudes in remote places, away from cities and pollution. The cultivated reishi is highly standardised, so you know you're getting the key medicinal ingredients.

Cultivation is often done by grafting spores on to Duanmu logs or on to Japanese oak. The Mayuzumi family in Japan, for example, have been cultivating reishi for over 25 years. The logs are placed in long rows in greenhouses and covered in wood crumbs and kept under strict environmental controls. The mushrooms are harvested after the sporing period. This can also be done in the wild, and there are many farms high in the mountains that produce natural and sustainable semi-wild reishi away from pollutants, using clean spring water and absolutely no chemicals.

There have been recorded side effects from taking reishi for over two months, including headaches, a dry mouth, stomach aches and dizziness. Please do work with a trained practitioner if you have any concerns over your health, and if you experience side effects stop taking reishi immediately.

It is recommended that vitamin C is taken alongside reishi in order to reap the full medicinal effects.

1. Grow Your Own

Many companies offer log growing kits. Look for companies that are Soil Association approved and organic. Maesyffin Mushrooms in West Wales are an award-wining organic shiitake-growing company and there are companies like this in most countries.

2. Reishi Spore Oil

If the thought of the mushroom itself doesn't inspire then consider the oil, which is believed to be more potent than the mushroom.

The hard spores are released from the underside of the body of the mushroom and cover it in its entirety, and contain an oil that's rich in triterpenes. In order to harvest this medicinal oil the spores are 'cracked' and the oil collected and put into capsules to be taken as a supplement. It is available from companies such as Dragon Herbs.

3. Reishi Tea

Reishi contains a carbohydrate called chitin which makes it very tough, so in order to penetrate the medicinal molecules you'll need to make a decoction that will allow the release of the beneficial water-soluble polysaccharides.

Use around a tablespoonful of small broken or sliced mushrooms to five cups of water and place these in a non-aluminum, preferably ceramic, pot on your stove.

Bring the water to the boil with the lid on and once boiling, reduce the heat and simmer for at least two hours. Remove from the heat and strain.

You should have enough to set aside and reheat for later, or you can store in the fridge for a few days to take each day. Drink 2–3 cups daily.

If it's too bitter you can add honey or other sweet tonic herbs such as sarsaparilla or ginger. You can also let the tea cool and add to broths and stews, or drink as your morning juice or smoothie, or made into a syrup.

4. Reishi Hug

This tonic drink is packed with antioxidants.

1 cup of nut milk (e.g. cashew milk)
½ tablespoon of linseeds
½ tablespoon of flaxseeds
½ teaspoon of chia seeds
1 tablespoon of coconut oil
1 tablespoon of honey
½ cup of dates
1 teaspoon of turmeric (page 249)
1 teaspoon of reishi powder
¼ teaspoon of ginger powder (page 81)

Simply blend all the ingredients and drink!

5. Satisfying Breakfast Smoothie

A nourishing breakfast in itself.

1 banana (or chopped frozen banana)
1 teaspoon of hemp seeds
1 teaspoon of cocoa nibs
1 teaspoon of reishi powder
1 teaspoon of rose hip powder
1 cup of blueberries
1 tablespoon of honey
1 cup of cashew nut milk

Blend everything together and serve.

6. Reishi Smoothie

This smoothie makes a good way to start the day if feeling exhausted and stressed.

½ an avocado
1 cup of spinach
1 thumb-sized piece of ginger (page 81)
1 cup of blueberries
½ cup of goji berries
1 teaspoon of reishi powder
1 teaspoon of astragalus powder (page 29)

Blend all the ingredients and enjoy!

7. Mushroom Stir Fry

This veggie stir fry makes an immune-boosting, supporting dish for the whole family. Serve with a side dish of rice if you like.

Serves 4

Oil for frying
1 shallot, chopped
2 cloves of garlic, crushed
1 carrot, sliced
A handful of kale
A whole broccoli head, chopped
A handful of button mushrooms
A handful of shiitake mushrooms
2 tablespons of nori seaweed flakes
2 teaspoons of reishi powder

Add the shallot and garlic to a frying pan with a little oil and fry gently.

Add the carrot, kale, broccoli and mushrooms and cook until soft. Sprinkle on the seaweed flakes and reishi and stir.

Season with salt and a little Nutty Salad Topping from the Gotu Kola chapter (see page 100), if you like.

8. Hot Chocolate with Reishi

This may sound like an odd mixture but the ingredients work together perfectly to make a warming, comforting drink.

Serves 2

500ml of nut milk (I prefer almond milk)
½ teaspoon of reishi powder
2 teaspoons of raw cacao powder
Pinch of sea salt
Pinch of cinnamon
1 tablespoon of coconut butter

Simmer the nut milk in a pan on the stove. Meanwhile, mix the remaining ingredients in a blender. Add the warmed milk to the blender and pulse through a few times until all the ingredients are mixed. Pour and drink.

9. Chest Supporter

Reishi supports chronic chest complaints and allergies. This recipe is a twist on the well-known onion cough syrup which does the same.

A jar of good quality honey (try manuka for its digestive-supporting
  properties)
6 teaspoons of reishi powder
1 onion, sliced lengthways
A 200ml Kilner jar

Mix the honey with the reishi powder. Layer the onion on the
bottom of the jar and then add a spoonful of honey. Keep adding
onion slices and then the honey until the jar is full.

Leave overnight or for up to 12 hours. Take a few spoonfuls of
the honey every 3 hours and keep in the fridge for up to 2 days.

10. Reishi Tincture

This is an easy, convenient way to take your reishi daily.

A cup of sliced or shredded reishi
500ml of good brandy or vodka
500ml airtight jar
150ml bottles

Place the reishi in a sterilised dry glass jar, filling it about
two-thirds full. Pour over the alcohol, making sure the reishi is
completely covered. Place the lid on and store in a cool, dry, dark
place for a few weeks. Shake the bottle gently every few days.

After a few weeks, strain the tincture into a bowl using a fine
sieve or some muslin. Pour the tincture into amber bottles and
don't forget to label and date them. This should keep for a few
years.

You can find a reishi tincture from a reputable herbal company
such as Fushi or Nature's Answer.

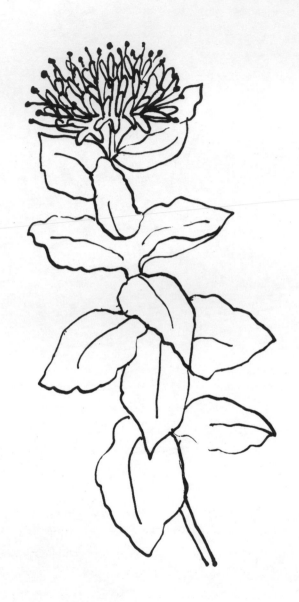

Rhodiola

Rhodiola rosea

Native to: Europe, Asia, North America

My favourite uses: to boost fertility, as protection from emotional environmental and physical stressors, for depression

Rhodiola belongs to the sedum or orpine family and is also known as rose root, because of its rose-smelling roots, and Arctic rose root because of its native location in the northern hemisphere. A good quality root extract should have the scent of rose because of its geraniol oil content, which gives the rose its fragrance.

This hardy perennial loves high altitudes with a dry, sandy soil and grows up to 75cm tall with thick succulent leaves and a round cluster of small yellow or pink flowers at the top.

Rhodiola is a superherb that helps support us through environmental, physical and emotional stress. It's thought to be superior to ginseng when suffering extreme stress, and it helps us metabolise serotonin, the 'happy hormone'.

It has been tested and used by Russian athletes to enhance

performance, both mentally and physically, and to improve their recovery times. It restores immune function, balances blood sugar, energises the body to help lessen fatigue, and enhances fertility in both men and women.

The Greek physician Dioscorides first documented this plant, which he called *Rodia riza*, in his medical text *De Materia Medica* in the first century AD. Carl Linnaeus, the famous Swedish botanist and taxonomist, renamed it *Rhodiola rosea* because of its rose-like fragrance. He noted its use for headaches and hysteria in his *Materia Medica* of 1749.

It is believed to have been used long ago by the Vikings, who probably discovered this adaptogen in Iceland and possibly chewed on its root to give themselves stamina and strength during their long journeys at sea.

In Siberia the roots of the rhodiola are part of the inhabitants' history and culture, and it was believed that you would live for a hundred years if it was taken every day. Strong decoctions of the root have been taken for centuries to help people cope with the harsh environment. It symbolised health and fertility and the roots were given to couples before their wedding night. It was also taken regularly to help alleviate fatigue, digestive problems and nervous exhaustion, and its whereabouts in its native habitat, harvesting and preserving techniques were closely guarded secrets within the community.

The Mongolians used rhodiola in the treatment of tuberculosis, pneumonia and cancer, and for preventing illness in the long winter months. Tibetan monks took a decoction to help calm their mind for meditation, and Sherpas used the root to help oxygenate the blood while trekking at high altitudes.

Rhodiola in traditional Chinese medicine dates back centuries, and is known as *hong jing tian*. It is used to replenish *qi* or *chi* energy, supporting heart and spleen function, boosting mental focus, clearing the lungs, calming the nervous system and strengthening the immune system. It is also used in TCM by those suffering from general weakness and exhaustion and for support after an illness or chronic disease.

Today it is grown beyond the Artic regions, from Iceland, Sweden and Asia to the Pyrenees and the Alps and the northern mountains of Canada and Alaska. Since the 1960s rhodiola has been one of the most researched adaptogens thanks to the Soviet Union, because of the plant's ability to enhance both mental and physical performance. Rhodiola helped the Soviets compete against the West in industry, sport, space travel and the military. It was officially registered in the Russian *Pharmacopoeia* in 1969 as an adaptogen that would help increase physical endurance and help overcome fatigue and stress.

Rhodiola contains many active substances of various terpenoids, flavonoids, phenols and alkaloids. The most important therapeutic effects are from the primary active compounds, rosavins and salidroside, which are unique to *Rhodiola rosea*. These active compounds are believed to affect the central nervous system to increase concentration and enhance stamina, acting as a natural antidepressant and anxiety reliever.

The growing popularity of this herb has meant that there has been over-harvesting in many countries, as most rhodiola today derives from plants collected in the wild. One-quarter of the rootstock should remain in the ground, and it should not be possible to harvest again from this portion for another 8–10 years. Consequently *Rhodiola rosea* has been on the rare plants list in Siberia since the 1980s. In order to protect this species, try to buy from reputable organically cultivated, sustainably harvested sources. Your supplier should state this clearly.

How Rhodiola Can Benefit You

Important note

Although it acts as a stimulant, this cooling adaptogen does not cause overstimulation of the nervous system. But if you have a strong sensitivity to stimulating foods please consult a qualified herbal practitioner or doctor before use.

Rhodiola works as a helpful tonic to rebalance the body's vital force by supporting the whole body system. It helps us to age positively by keeping the body feeling calm, focused, strong and nourished, especially when confronted with life's stressors that have a negative effect on mood, sleep patterns, poor or over-active appetite and exhaustion.

The key constituent in rhodiola is salidroside, a glucoside which has been shown to have neuroprotective, anti-cancer and antidepressant potential.

Mind

This is a beneficial adaptogen for those high achievers who overwork the body and the mind.

The stress hormone cortisol can also impede mental clarity and make the mind wander; rhodiola helps to balance the adrenals, helping to manage stress more positively. When we experience constant emotional and/or physical stress, cortisol is released into our system which, over a long period of time, can have a damaging effect on our nervous system, metabolic system, immune system, and cardiovascular system, affecting our whole well-being and our ageing process.

Memory tests have shown that rhodiola helps to enhance concentration by reducing mental fatigue and increasing mental performance. It boosts the memory and the brain's learning capacity while decreasing mental fatigue or brain fog – a good adaptogen for students sitting exams at university or for those who sit for long periods at a computer.

The positive effects of rhodiola help to improve mood and relieve fatigue. It helps support mild to moderate depression, anxiety states and attention. The support of the nervous system and its ability to calm the mind make it a good remedy for ADD.

A clinical trial documented in the *Nordic Journal of Psychiatry* in 2007 carried out a double-blind placebo-controlled study on both men and women aged from 18 to 70 years who were assessed and selected for varying degrees of depression and separated into three groups. Two groups were given different doses of rhodiola extract and the third group a placebo and the participants were assessed over a 6-week period. The participants in both groups taking the rhodiola extract saw a significant improvement in overall depression, insomnia and emotional instability, but not in self-esteem; whereas the placebo group showed no improvement. There were no side effects reported and the conclusion was that rhodiola shows definite anti-depressive potency in patients with mild to moderate depression.

Body

Rhodiola helps to increase the body's ability to utilise energy from the body's cells more efficiently, helping with feelings of fatigue and exhaustion and supporting the body with improved sleep patterns.

It is used to increase strength and endurance and shorten recovery time after prolonged physical activity by athletes. It is also believed to help burn fat quicker and lessens any muscle stiffness after exertion.

Cardiac problems caused by stress, such as arrhythmias, have been found to be supported by rhodiola, which helps to improve the overall action of the heart muscle.

Its high antioxidant content makes rhodiola a good cancer preventative by reducing oxidative damage from free radicals.

It is believed to have a balancing effect on the thyroid, enhancing and balancing thyroid function in mild hypothyroidism without over-stimulating the gland and causing hyperthyroidism.

It improves sexual function in both men and women who are suffering from exhaustion and depression.

Beauty and Spirit

Emotional and physical stress takes its toll on our skin, as do environmental pollutants. Rhodiola's ability to protect the body from all of these makes our skin less susceptible to premature ageing. Rhodiola is a new ingredient that is being used by the beauty industry because of its high concentration of antioxidants to counteract the effects of pollution, and UV sun damage that is incredibly ageing.

When used specifically for the skin rhodiola has been found to boost circulation, and stimulate the production of collagen, helping to keep the skin supple and reducing fine lines.

Rhodiola is used to replenish *qi* or *chi* energy, the life force helping to reconnect us with ourselves and rejuvenate our spirit.

Ten Ways with Rhodiola

As with most adaptogens, rhodiola's benefits build up over a period of regular use. The root is used medicinally and is a little bitter and very drying, tasting of a mixture of roses and oranges combined.

Try to take this balancing herb a few weeks before travelling and during the journey to support the body through the stresses of modern travel, especially flights.

As mentioned before, please try to buy from organic suppliers or from sustainably harvested sources, to encourage wild rhodiola to flourish.

1. Coconut Breakfast Drink

To stave off adrenal exhaustion and stop that 'hitting the wall' feeling in times of stress at home or at work, try this in the morning as your go-to alternative for a quick, nutritious and supportive breakfast.

1 teaspoon of rhodiola powder
1 teaspoon of bee pollen (page 39)
1 teaspoon of pine pollen
4 teaspoons of manuka honey
1 tablespoon of coconut butter
1 teaspoon of matcha blended into a cup of warm water
400ml of good quality raw coconut milk

Place all of the above into a blender and blend for just 2–3 pulses until frothy.

2. Rhodiola Latte

This caffeine-free latte makes a warming beverage at any time of day. Bee pollen gives an added antioxidant hit.

2 teaspoons of rhodiola powder
1 teaspoon of turmeric powder (page 249)
1 cup of almond milk (or milk of choice)
1 dessertspoon of good quality honey
2 teaspoons of bee pollen (page 39)

Place the rhodiola and turmeric in a mug. Simmer the milk and pour a little into the bottom of the mug, whisking with a fork or whisk so the herbs blend. Add the remaining milk and then sprinkle a couple of teaspoons of bee pollen and honey for flavour and an extra health boost.

3. Fruit Juice with a Difference

If you like making your own fruit juices give this one a try.

1 cup of strawberries
1 cup of raspberries
½ cup of red currants
½ cup of blackcurrants
2 teaspoons of rhodiola powder
1 teaspoon of freeze dried goji berry powder

Blend or slow press the berries and currants. Add the herb powders, drink and feel the buzz.

4. Mind-focusing Drink

When suffering from brain fog, an over-stressed mind, or when you just can't think straight, support the mind with this healthy drink.

1 teaspoon of rhodiola powder
1 teaspoon of reishi powder (page 181)
2 teaspoon of gotu kola herb, made into a 110ml infusion
175g of raw coconut cream
3 teaspoons of raw honey

Blend all of the above and enjoy.

5. Veggie Soup

This light soup makes a great way to get your 5-a-day.

Serves 2

4 spring onions, chopped
3 cloves of garlic, chopped
Coconut oil for frying
1 cup of shiitake mushrooms, fresh if possible, sliced
1 bunch of asparagus (400g), trimmed
1 thumb-sized piece of fresh ginger, peeled and sliced
1.2 litres of organic vegetable stock
2 teaspoons of soya paste
Sweet soya sauce
200g of fresh organic washed spinach leaves
2 teaspoons of powdered rhodiola

Soften the spring onion and garlic in a little coconut oil in a heavy bottomed, non-aluminium saucepan.

Add the mushrooms, asparagus, ginger and stock and simmer for 10 minutes.

Then add the soya paste and a few shakes of sweet soya sauce. Finally add the spinach and let this wilt. Stir in the rhodiola powder and serve.

6. Rhodiola Honey

This honey makes a delicious spread or stir through, and is an easy way of adding this herb into your daily diet.

4 tablespoons of powdered rhodiola root
A pot manuka or thyme honey

Clean and sterilise a small jar. Place the rhodiola powder in the bottom and add a good quality medicinal honey, stirring to mix the powder with the honey.

Spread on toast or add to your warm infusions for a little extra stress-relieving support.

7. Refreshing and Stress-relieving Infusion

A delicious and refreshing blend, full of antioxidants and with a distinct flavour.

50g of dried rhodiola root or 2 teaspoons of rhodiola powder
A small handful of dried rose petals or buds
½ cup of wild pine pollen from hybrid herbs (you can find this
  online or at Planet Organic)
½ cup of dried spearmint or peppermint leaves

Place all of the ingredients in a blender and blend for just a few pulses.

Put in an airtight container. Use 1 teaspoon to a cup of boiling water and allow to infuse for 15 minutes.

Breathe in the soothing, refreshing aroma as it cools and infuses, then sip.

8. Tonic Decoction

This decoction helps to maintain stamina and balance.

1.2 litres of filtered water
1 cup of dried rose hips (page 209)
2 strips of astragalus root (page 29)
1 teaspoon of rhodiola dried root
A little liquorice root (page 143)
A thumb-sized piece of fresh ginger (page 81)

Add all of the ingredients to a heavy pan (not an aluminium one), and simmer with the lid on (to keep in the essential oils) for 20 minutes. Do not heat for any longer as the rhodiola can become quite astringent and bitter.

Add honey to taste and drink every day when feeling exhausted and overwhelmed.

9. Easy Rhodiola Tincture

½ cup of dried rhodiola root, sliced
500ml of good quality vodka or brandy

Add the rhodiola root slices to a bottle until it is about two-thirds full. Then add the alcohol, keeping a few centimetres free at the top of the bottle neck.

Place the top on and keep it somewhere safe away from direct sunlight and heat for 3 weeks. The alcohol acts as a solvent for all the therapeutic constituents of the rhodiola.

After 3 weeks strain the herb from the tincture and rebottle. It should keep for around 3 years.

Drink 10–20 drops in a little water every day.

10. Rhodiola and Rose Petal Salve for Sun Damage

Use this to soothe irritated and inflamed sun-damaged skin.

6 teaspoons of rhodiola powder
50g of rose petals
225ml of olive oil
25g of beeswax
20 drops of rose geranium essential oil

Place the herbs in a bain-marie (see page 26) with the olive oil and simmer for 3 hours. Then strain the herbs through muslin and keep the oil.

Place the infused oil back in the bain-marie. Add the beeswax and heat until the wax melts into the oil. Turn off the heat and add the rose geranium essential oil.

Pour into salve tins to store. They should be labelled and dated and they should last for about 1 year.

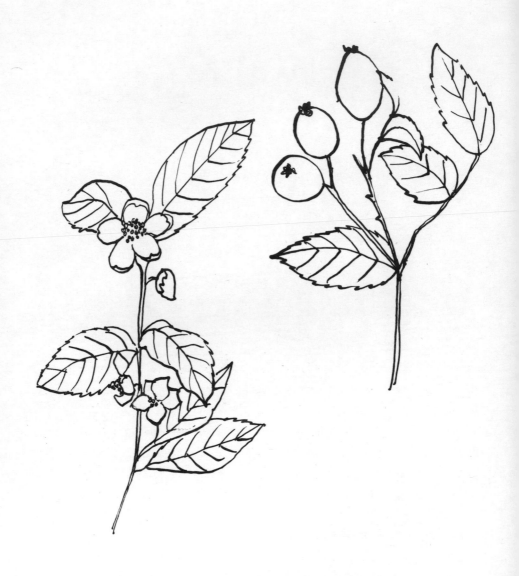

Rose Hips

Rosa canina

Native to: Europe, Asia and West Africa

My favourite uses: for colds and flu, building the immune system, lack of vitality, convalescing, as an anti-inflammatory

Roses are a beautiful deciduous shrub known universally as a symbol of love. Their scent is captivating and uplifting to our spirits. They are known to 'raise the spirits and cheer the heart'; in bloom they act as a mild sedative, an antidepressant, antiviral and an aphrodisiac. But when the fragrance has gone and the petals have fallen, the nutritious fruit of the rose known as the rose hip continues to nourish and balance us ... the rose just keeps on giving.

You may be familiar with rose hips, the shiny red fruits that appear when the petals of the rose flower fall after their bloom in early Autumn, but you probably would not expect them to be included as an adaptogen herb. However, the *Rosa* species has been found to have the ability to boost the immune system while calming and strengthening the nervous system, balancing the whole body system.

There are suggestions that rose hips were a staple source of food, along with hawthorn, when food was scarce from the Iron Age onwards. Before any understanding of what vitamin C was or of its actions, people would use and prescribe rose hips when suffering from a cold, flu, inflammation or bleeding gums. Pliny the Elder records their use in the first century AD. The rose has been used throughout the centuries for medicine, in foods, perfumery, cloth dying and ritual.

Native American women would use rose hips as part of their daily winter food, drinking the water used to soften them, then adding the stewed fruit as an accompaniment to meals. Dried rose hips were also used for nourishment in the long hard winter months. Medicinally, the hips, petals and leaves were used in cases of flu, stomach upsets and fever.

In traditional Chinese medicine the rose hip has been used for centuries to rebalance the kidney energy and for urinary incontinence. The astringency of the rose hip has made it useful in cases of chronic diarrhoea in both TCM and Ayurvedic medicine.

The hips of the *Rosa rugose*, which have larger tomato-shaped hips, and the sweet briar rose, *Rosa rubiginosa*, can both be used medicinally, but it is the dog rose, *Rosa canina*, thought to have derived its name from its use in healing dog bites in the Roman era, that is most often used medicinally.

Native to Europe, Asia and West Africa the dog rose can be found growing in thickets and hedgerows. It can also be cultivated – we had many in our garden when I was little. It has a beautiful and delicate white pinkish rose with a summery fragrance, and thorny branches that can reach to over 3 metres.

In Britain during the Second World War, the government encouraged everyone to return to foraging to supplement the food ration. The Ministry of Food published advice on how to forage with the help of Herb Committees set up across the nation for the 'Hedgerow Harvest', which focused mainly on the nutritious and versatile rose hip. Nationally everyone was at risk of vitamin C deficiency, especially young children, due to a shortage of fresh vegetables and citrus fruits. Rose hips were collected on an enormous scale – arranged through schools, boy scout and girl guide groups and the Women's Institute, with 2 shillings given for every 14lb collected. Commercially appointed companies then made some 134 million rose hips into 600,000 bottles of syrup. There was even a National Rose Hip Syrup Day when the syrup went on sale on 1 February 1941.

How Rose Hips Can Benefit You

Rose hips are an impressive immune-system booster. I use these natural jewels in a syrup during our long damp winter months here in England, when I feel there is a need for extra protection from recurring colds, flu and tummy bugs. Hips contain one of the highest natural plant sources of vitamin C available – as much as 20 per cent more than citrus fruit, weight for weight. And it's much easier for the body to assimilate than synthetic vitamin C supplements commonly used to build resistance over the winter period. Rose hips support immunity, they detox the system, and they are cooling, making them a good remedy for flu and colds.

To harvest the hips, wait until after the first frosts, when the hips are a vibrant, beautiful, shiny ripe red – then they're ready for picking. Please note that the traditional cultivated rose hips from roses found in parks and gardens have a lot fewer medicinal and nutritional benefits than wild roses, and often have been sprayed with pesticides.

Mind

Rose hips lighten the mood, helping to reduce anxiety and mild depression. They support the nervous system when feeling overwhelmed and run down. In the elderly and those recovering from an illness they help to improve resistance and health – and also promote a more positive outlook.

Rose hips nourish and support with their adaptogenic effect. They help to calm and support an exhausted nervous system while being uplifting and strengthening to the mind and spirit.

Body

Rose hips contain antioxidants, carotenoids, polyphenols, flavonoids, plant sterols and essential fatty acids, which make them not just an impressive immune-system booster, giving the body protection from the common cold virus, but also they work hard for you as a cancer preventative.

The main constituents of the rose hip are also believed to help support the function of the cardiovascular system, helping to prevent heart disease by inhibiting the oxidation of LDL low density lipoproteins, or so-called 'bad' cholesterol.

They also help the digestive system by acting as a nourishing and gentle natural laxative, as well as reducing painful spasms in cases of diarrhoea. They have been found to be gently toning to the gall bladder too, which helps with digestion of fats.

To help maintain a balanced kidney energy include rose hips in your diet. In traditional Chinese medicine, the kidneys are seen as the vital force of the whole body, supplying energy to those organs needing assistance and running on empty. Rose hips help prevent the formation of gravel and kidney stones (especially in those who are susceptible), and act as a mild diuretic for those needing to expel excess fluid from the body in case of water retention and oedema. Overall, rose hips are just a general incredible kidney tonic.

They have an anti-allergic effect on the system, with their high antioxidant content making them super beneficial if you are a seasonal hay fever sufferer or have allergic rhinitis.

Rose hips have also been found to be anti-inflammatory and a proven pain reliever. A study of 300 patients suffering from osteo-arthritis gave them different pain relief and rose hip powder made from the fruits and husks over a 3-month period. The published results from the Frederiksberg Hospital in Copenhagen were astounding: rose hip powder was found to be three times more effective for pain relief than paracetamol, and 40 per cent more effective than using a glucosamine therapy, a natural constituent of cartilage. Other clinical trials were done on reducing pain in hip osteoarthritis and chronic knee pain and the results again were very positive. Rose hip not only reduces the pain without any of the negative side effects of conventional pain relief, but works to allay the inflammation that is associated with osteoarthritis.

Beauty and Spirit

I use rose hip oil in a hydrating herbal body oil that I like to formulate with herbs and essential oils for the skin. Hips are an amazingly rich source of calcium, silica, phosphorus and mag-nesium and, with their fatty acids and high levels of vitamin C and A, these nutrients not only help with cell renewal and anti-ageing – they also help heal the skin where there may be scarring from wounds or burns, stretch marks and sun damage.

The astringency of rose hip water works really well with acne and problem skin.

I'd recommend drinking an infusion of dried rose hips daily to keep your skin youthful and vibrant. Hips also help the body maintain its skin collagen – a protein that holds individual cells together and often touted by cosmetic companies because, as we get older, our bodies produce less.

Not bad from this amazing, free-to-forage fruit!

Ten Ways with Rose Hips

It's a good idea to remove the fine bristly hairs on the end of the hips before using them, as they can be irritating to the throat if they get stuck. You can remove the seeds as well, by cutting the hips in half and shaking out the seeds or removing them with your thumb, but this does take time. It can be a meditative practice though, with music playing!

If this is too much however, try putting the whole hips in a pan, cover with water and simmer for about 50 minutes. Then remove from the heat and strain through a fine sieve. Rub the hips through as much as you can, leaving the pulp, hairs and seeds and keeping the juice.

You can use the juice for the recipes below or you can freeze it for later use. The whole hip freezes really well too.

1. Drying Rose Hips

It is useful to know how to dry rose hips so that you can use them at a later date when they are not in season.

Collect enough rose hips that you can store. Try to pick the deep red hips and leave the orange ones to ripen more for later picking.

Go through the hips to remove the ones that are mouldy or rotten. Give them a good wash and place them on a tea towel to dry. Then lay them out on a baking sheet, parchment paper or drying sheets – if you have one, use a dehydrator . . . this may take just a few hours.

Leave the hips in a dark, dry, well-ventilated safe place for a few weeks. They should go wrinkly and darker and feel harder to touch after this time. Then place in a clean, dry, airtight container, and store away from direct sunlight to always have the nutritional benefits of rose hip to hand.

If you need to rehydrate your hips, leave them to soak in water overnight.

2. Breakfast Hips for Cereal

With all the expensive packaged powders and seeds on the market made specifically to add to cereals and smoothies, I thought it may be inspiring – and cheaper – to make your own.

Place 500g of dried rose hips in a blender or food processor and grind or pulse a few times until you have ground berries, but not too powdered.

Then pour the rose hips into a small sieve and shake into a clean bowl, allowing the hairs and any hard, unpalatable bits to come away from your hips. The seeds are fine left in.

Place the ground hips in a clean, dry, airtight container and sprinkle on cereal or add to a smoothie with your super greens and bee pollen.

3. Decoction of Rose Hips

This is such a good way to keep the immune system vital and also to actively heal yourself when full of a cold or flu.

Place 3 teaspoons of fresh (clean) or dried rose hips, sliced, in a small saucepan with 3 cups of filtered water. Bring to the boil, and then simmer for 15 minutes.

Pour into a cup and add honey to taste.

4. Rose Hip Soup

This is a Swedish favourite called *Nyponsoppa* which dates back
to when foraging for rose hips was done in the long, harsh winter
months, before foods became available out of season, flown in
from countries around the world. Swedes would collect the rose
hips and prepare this soup as a starter or dessert to ensure they
had the essential nutrients they needed to keep their immune
systems strong.

Serves 2

About 5 cups of ripe rose hips
8 cups of filtered water
½ cup of granulated sugar
1 teaspoon of cornflour

Cut each hip in half and remove the hairs and seeds.

Put the prepared hips in a saucepan with the water. Bring to
the boil and then simmer for 45 minutes. Cook until the hips
are soft, giving the liquid a chance to reduce.

Take off the heat and put the liquid into a food processor or
blender and pulse a few times. Strain the mashed hips through
muslin or a fine sieve back into the pan. Add the sugar and put
the pan on to simmer again. Discard the strained pulp.

Blend the cornflour with a little hot water to form a soft paste,
and add the paste a little at a time to the pan, stirring continuously until the soup thickens slightly.

Serve hot or cold. I like to add a sprig of fresh mint, basil or
chervil to garnish. Traditionally a little crème fraiche or cream
was added.

5. Fresh Rose Hip and Blackberry Jam

This jam is packed full of antioxidants and is easy to make.

Enjoy picking your fresh rose hips and blackberries. Then give your fruit a good wash and leave to dry wrapped in a tea cloth.

Take the rose hips and discard all the mouldy and bruised ones. Place the rest in a pan and pour in water until they're just covered. Simmer for about 30–40 minutes, stirring and mashing with a wooden spoon at intervals until the hips are soft.

Push the mashed-up rose hips through a fine sieve, collecting all the juice and flesh in a bowl and leaving the hairs and seeds in the sieve.

Weigh the rosehip mash and the blackberries and put back into the pan. Add the equivalent weight in sugar to this fruit mash, and the juice of a lemon.

Bring to a slow boil till the consistency is sticky like jam … this usually takes around 15 minutes. Turn off the heat and spoon your jam into sterilised airtight jam jars. Label and date the jars.

6. Rose Hip Syrup

This is really delicious on yoghurt with seasonal fresh berries, or diluted as a cordial for kids. It's a recipe you have to repeat twice, which may sound laborious but it is actually really easy.

Makes about 1 litre of syrup

1litre of filtered water
500g of fresh berries, washed, with the bruised and mouldy ones
  removed
250g of soft brown sugar or coconut sugar (which has a lower
  glycaemic index because of its inulin content, a fibre that acts as
  a prebiotic feeding the good bacteria of the gut)

Bring half the water to the boil.

Chop your rose hips in half or pulse them in the food processor once or twice. Add the hips to the boiling water and simmer gently for 20 minutes.

Pour the contents of your pan into a jelly bag or through a fine muslin cloth and allow the juice to drip through. This should take 20–30 minutes. Help this process along a little by gently squeezing and pushing the pulp through.

Put the sieved pulp and juice back into the pan again with the rest of the water and bring this back to the boil, repeating the same process as before. Strain through the jelly bag or through fine muslin cloth and allow the juice to drip through again.

Put the juice back into the pan and simmer gently. Add the sugar and stir continuously until all the sugar has dissolved.

Pour the hot liquid into a sterilised Kilner clip-top bottle, label and date. It should keep for 3 months in the fridge.

7. Rose Hip Vinegar

This is a soothing remedy as a gargle for sore throats. Or mixed with hot water and honey for easing colds and flu.

A few cups of rose hips
500ml (or the size of your container) of a good quality apple cider vinegar

Slit a few cupfuls of freshly selected, cleaned and dried rose hips and place them in a 500ml Kilner jar. Cover with a good quality apple cider vinegar.

Leave to infuse on a window ledge in a sunny spot for 4–6 weeks. Then strain and rebottle the infused rose hip vinegar.

Mix a tablespoon into a little warm water for a gargle, and into a cup of water for a hot infusion with honey. You could add thyme to give it more of an antiviral, antibacterial kick.

You can use it in salad dressings too.

8. Rose Hip Oxymel

An oxymel, from the Latin meaning acid and honey, is a herbal preparation made with just that: vinegar and honey. They were once a popular way of taking herbs and are really very tasty. This should store well for up to 3 months.

A few cups of fresh rose hips, cleaned and cut in half
Apple cider vinegar, preferably organic
Good quality honey

Place the clean rose hips in a tall sterilised jam jar. They should fill it a quarter full.

Add equal amounts of apple cider vinegar and honey until the jar is full. (I like to use infused honey, such as elderflower, to add to the immune-boosting properties.) Place the lid on, sealing the jar.

Shake the jar and then leave somewhere in a safe dark spot for 2 weeks, shaking the jar gently every few days. After 2 weeks, strain and pour into another jar and seal, label and date.

Take a dessertspoonful every few hours to help get you back on your feet during the flu or a cold.

9. My Cedar, Patchouli and Rose Hip Body Oil

This heals and protects the skin – and lifts the spirits. Store out of direct sunlight and use within 3 months of making.

30ml of jojoba oil
20ml of rose hip oil
20ml of calendula oil
10ml of vitamin E oil
20 drops of cedar essential oil
15 drops of patchouli essential oil

Mix the above together in a beaker and pour into 100ml amber bottle with pump or pipette.

Use on damp skin after a shower to rehydrate and soothe the skin.

10. Hip Hand Balm

This is a rich skin-nourishing treatment your hands will love. It should last for 6–12 months.

20g of shea butter
5g of beeswax
20ml of jojoba oil
20ml of rose hip oil
A few fresh wild rose petals (optional)
5ml of vitamin E oil
5 drops of rose essential oil
15 drops of frankincense essential oil
10 drops of clary sage essential oil

Take a saucepan, quarter fill with water and place an aluminium bowl in the top so that it rests above the water, making a bain-marie.

Bring the water to a gentle boil and add the shea butter and beeswax to the bowl and stir gently till melted.

Then add the jojoba and rose hip oil (and rose petals, if

using), mixing until blended. Then remove from the heat and stir in the vitamin E oil to preserve your balm and the essential oils.

Pour into balm tins and leave them to cool before screwing on the lid.

After washing hands, apply enough to your fingers to massage into the backs of your hands.

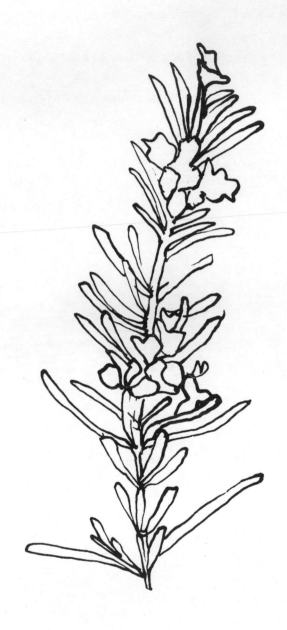

Rosemary

Rosmarinus

Native to: the Mediterranean and Asia

My favourite uses: for the elderly, strengthening memory and the brain's vitality, chronic fatigue, emotional upset

This wonderful well-known fragrant aromatic herb belongs to the mint family Lamiaceae. The name *rosmarinus* comes from the Latin meaning 'dew of the sea' and it is native to the Mediterranean region. Like most adaptogens, rosemary is a hardy plant that manages to adapt to live well in the most difficult conditions.

Its small, tough, needle-shaped leaves, which are rich in volatile oil, are the parts used for its medicinal purpose, and they are at their most potent when the whole plant is flowering in the spring and summer months – or maybe all year round in temperate climes.

Rosemary is one of the first herbs I had knowledge of as a child. Rosemary, lavender and mint grew freely around our garden and I loved making potions by crushing the fragrant leaves. My mum only used it as a culinary herb, but the smell of rosemary rubbed between my fingers, and the rich aroma as it roasted in the oven, will always remind me of my childhood and home.

Auspiciously, when rosemary is planted at the entrance of your home, it is believed to protect all who live there. My window boxes are planted with rosemary for their culinary and healing use and for their extra protection ... it also generally takes care of itself.

Traditionally rosemary was used in a bride's wedding bouquet, and in the wreaths at funerals in the Victorian period as a symbol of remembrance. Lovers would give a sprig to one another as a sign of their fidelity.

Rosemary is rich in antioxidants such as phenolic acid and rosemarinic acid. Rosemarinic acid is a very powerful antioxidant, antiviral and an anti-inflammatory. Phenolic acid helps the body utilise vitamin E, increasing its antioxidant potential. Most of the other antioxidants contained in rosemary have been shown to potentially inhibit ageing symptoms of the brain.

How Rosemary Can Benefit You

Look on rosemary as a rejuvenating and stimulating adaptogen. It acts as one of the more gentle adaptogen herbs, but still works wonders to support the whole body system, helping to strengthen endurance, calm our nervous system, and lifting our spirits both mentally and physically.

The first herbal book to be printed in England in 1525, known as the *Bankes' Herbal* after its author, held of rosemary that '*to smell the scent of the leaves kept one youngly*'.

Mind

Rosemary is known as the 'herb of remembrance' and it works as a perfect tonic for the brain. It strengthens the capillaries and increases blood circulation to the brain, stimulating brain function and increasing concentration and memory. This makes the herb perfect for the elderly to help them achieve healthy ageing, and for those needing extra help with brain power, such as city workers, lawyers, doctors and those still learning.

Rosemary helps with our overall positive mental outlook, helping those suffering from anxiety and depression. It is also a perfect remedy for tension and emotional headaches, and headaches due to overindulgence.

Body

Rosemary supports the whole nervous system, acting as a tonic for nervous tension and helping relieve lethargy and exhaustion, calming and soothing the central nervous system and helping to relieve insomnia. It is a wonderful herb for those suffering from chronic fatigue syndrome.

Rosemary's high antioxidant content helps to protect the whole body from the ill effects of ageing. Its warming and stimulating properties get the blood moving, which makes this aromatic herb a perfect choice for those who need more vitality and vigour, strengthening the heart and helping protect the arteries from arteriosclerosis.

It works well to get the body's circulation moving to the peripheries, supporting the heart and warming the hands and feet. Externally its stimulating action is of great benefit to those who feel the cold or suffer from Raynaud's disease and chilblains as a rub and foot bath.

The aromatic oils of rosemary help to stimulate a sluggish

digestion, stoking those 'digestive fires' to help those who suffer from dyspepsia, bloating and constipation. It also helps to allay cramping of the stomach and intestines with diarrhoea, acting as a calming astringent.

Rosemary has been shown to help support the liver, improving enzyme production and helping to lower blood glucose and cholesterol levels. It is also used by herbalists when there's an inflamed gall bladder and jaundice.

Use the aromatic oils of rosemary internally to help prevent infection and support the immune system, helping to relieve a sore throat and congestion, helping to clear phlegm where there's a cough and blocked sinus. Rosemary's a strong antibacterial, antiviral and antiseptic herb and it is really useful as an antiviral room spray, or kept in your bag for first aid for cuts, grazes, bites and stings. I make up a room spray when there are colds and flu in the house and use fresh rosemary when I make up a healing salve.

As a liniment or rub this aromatic analgesic herb massaged into joints and muscles is wonderful at easing aches and pains and in cases of rheumatism, arthritis and backache, relieving tension. And the scent will definitely work to uplift your spirit.

Beauty and Spirit

Rosemary has been used for generations in preparations for the hair and skin because of its astringent, stimulating and anti-ageing properties.

Rosemary helps to stimulate the blood supply to the scalp to help with hair loss, and has been used to darken hair for decades and give it a beautiful shine. It is also useful to remember that rosemary's very good at preventing and ridding the hair of head lice – the creatures hate the aromatic oils!

Ten Ways with Rosemary

1. Smudge Stick

Smudging (also known as saging, as sage is often used for its negative energy-clearing abilities) is a Native American tradition, a ritual that anoints and protects. It's a way for us to connect with the Earth and to Nature.

Smudge sticks are a good way of ceremoniously saying goodbye to the old and welcoming the new. They're also used to de-stress the body and put a full stop on a particularly eventful day. Rosemary has a very long history of use as a herb of purification and protection.

A smudge stick is prepared by placing the dried herbs together, tied or in a clay pot. They are then set alight and the smoke is wafted around the person or room. I like to do this when I've moved into a new home (together with placing salt and bread on the front doorstep, symbols of health and stability), and I use them sometimes to cleanse and change the energy in a room, or when a child has been sick with a virus.

Rosemary for protection
Mugwort for purification
Sage to clear negative energy
Lavender for calming

To make a smudge stick, take a few longish sprigs (15–17cm or so) of your chosen herbs. Bundle them together facing the same way and wrap string tightly round the bottom. Then start to wrap string up the herbs, bunching them together with a few centimetres space between the string up to the top of the herbs. When you reach the tip of the smudge stick, work your way back down again with the same spacing of the string.

Tie the two bits of string together at the base and leave to dry in a warm dry place or on a drying screen for a week.

To smudge, light the top of the smudge stick and, once it has a steady flame, blow it out until it is smoking. Put it in a fire safe bowl that will catch the ash. You can also move the smudge stick around a room or person and fan the smoke.

2. Rosemary and Thyme-infused Oil

This is an Italian-inspired idea and one that you can be inventive with and add your own personal flavour favourites, such as garlic, chilli, peppercorns and even lemon. It is my go-to oil when cooking fish, chicken or roasting vegetables.

3 sprigs of rosemary
A few small bunches of thyme
500ml of good quality olive oil
A Kilner clip-top bottle

I like using sprigs of fresh rosemary and thyme as the dried herbs just aren't as flavoursome. The thyme gives your oil extra antioxidant, antibacterial tonic benefits.

Rinse the herbs but make sure they are absolutely dry, otherwise the water will make your oil rancid. Try to gently crush the herbs in your fingers to allow the volatile oils to mix with your olive oil.

Place the herbs in the Kilner bottle and then heat your oil in a saucepan till just warm – not bubbling. Pour into the bottle to cover the herbs, and seal.

Store in a cool dry place for up to 2 weeks, then use in cooking or as a delicious dip for bread.

3. Roasted Fruit and Rosemary

This dish is extremely easy and is a lovely sweet breakfast, dessert or snack idea. A delicious way to inspire you to incorporate rosemary into your daily dishes.

5 peaches, or 10 plums
3 tablespoons of brown sugar, or coconut sugar, or clear honey
3–4 sprigs of fresh rosemary
2 tablespoons of water

Preheat the oven to 200°C/gas mark 6 and place 2 rosemary sprigs in the bottom of your roasting tray.

Cut the fruit in half and remove the stones. Place the fruit in the roasting tray cut side up.

Sprinkle the sugar of choice or honey over the fruit and add a rosemary sprig or two on top.

Add a couple of tablespoons of water to stop everything drying and burning at the bottom. Bake for 30 minutes, until the fruit is soft and syrupy. Remove from the oven and enjoy the contrasting flavours of the sweet fruit with the bitter rosemary.

4. Herb Salt

A packet of sea salt
2 dessertspoons of Himalayan salt
A sprig of fresh rosemary, leaves removed from the stalk
A few sprigs of thyme, leaves removed from the stalk
A few basil leaves
A few sprigs of parsley

Put all the ingredients in a food processor and pulse until everything is mixed and of a fine texture. It will look a bit wet, so place on a baking sheet to air dry for a few hours.

Transfer to an airtight container. It should keep indefinitely.

5. Brain-enhancing Infusion

This infusion is good for nourishing the brain, increasing mental alertness and vitality. It is also good for memory loss, and is a nerve tonic too.

1 tablespoon of dried gotu kola (page 95)
1 tablespoon of dried ginkgo
1 tablespoon of dried hawthorn leaf (page 117)
1 tablespoon of dried rosemary

All of these herbs can be bought from good herb suppliers. Please see page 263 for a recommended list.

Mix all the herbs together in a clean dry container and then add to an airtight jar. This should store well for up to a year.

To prepare an infusion use 1 teaspoon per cup, or 3 teaspoons to a pot. Pour over boiling water and allow to infuse for up to 10 minutes.

Try to have up to 3 cups per day.

6. Herbal Facial Steam

I love aromatic herbal facial steams for their healing properties, rebalancing and deeply cleansing my skin. This formula uses rosemary which is good for normal-to-oily skin, as it is quite astringent.

3 dessertspoons of dried calendula

2 dessertspoons of dried chamomile

1 dessertspoon of dried rosemary

Boil 500ml of water. Place the herbs in a heatproof bowl on a heatproof surface, pour in the water and stir. Quickly cover the bowl with a tea towel for 3 minutes to allow the herbs to infuse and for the water to cool slightly.

Then lean over the bowl, remove the cloth and drape a large towel over your head, covering the bowl too, and breathe in the steam. Let it penetrate your face and skin pores.

If it is too hot under the towel, keep popping your head out for air, or just raise the towel to allow cool air in.

I steam for about 5 minutes. Then I let my face cool for a while before going back under the towel again for 10 minutes or so.

After a steam gently pat your face dry with a clean towel and apply a moisturising cream.

7. Revitalising Face Oil

2 tablespoons of rose hip oil

1 dessertspoon of vitamin E oil

20 drops of rosemary essential oil

10 drops of rose absolute essential oil

A 50ml dropper bottle

Put the rose hip oil and vitamin E oil in a dry clean bowl, and then add the essential oils and mix well. Pour the face oil into the dropper bottle (it might be easier with a small funnel), put the lid on and give it a shake. Label and leave for a day so that the oils can mix.

Use the oil by placing a few drops on clean fingertips, rub your fingers together to create some warmth and then massage the oil all over your face and neck, making sure to avoid the eyes.

Store in the fridge for up to four months and use every morning for a cooling, revitalising, moisturising lift.

8. The Queen of Hungary's Facial Water

This beauty product, dating from around the fourteenth century, was reputed to have been made by the court alchemist to cure ailments and help to beautify the ageing Queen Elizabeth of Hungary. An alternative story holds that it was gypsies who formulated and sold the water as a cure-all.

The first recipes mainly contained rosemary and thyme in brandy, and the water was a sought-after herbal remedy and cologne by the likes of Charles V of France.

This astringent toner tightens and refreshes the complexion, leaving the skin clear and even, perfect for oily skin. It also makes a nourishing rinse for hair. As an eau de cologne, use brandy to infuse the herbs and not vinegar – it will smell much better.

1 part dried rosemary
1 part dried thyme
1 part dried mint
1 part dried sage
1 part dried lemon peel
2 parts dried calendula
2 parts dried rose petals
2 parts dried comfrey
Rose water
Rose geranium essential oil
Apple cider vinegar (brandy for a cologne)

Place the dried herbs in a wide-mouthed jar. Cover with vinegar/ brandy so that all of the herbs are submerged. Secure with a lid and leave for 3 weeks in a warm place.

After 3 weeks strain off the herbs. To each cup of the herbal infusion add half a cup of rose water. Add a few drops of rose geranium essential oil to add potency to the scent.

Use as a herbal toner after cleansing, and as a hair rinse after shampooing.

9. Stimulating and Healing Bath Soak

This bath soak relaxes the muscles and the mind. It also smells incredible. You can find the oils at Neal's Yard Remedies or at online herbal stockists such as The Organic Trading Company (see page 263).

500ml of Epsom salts
1 tablespoon of dried rosemary
½ tablespoon of dried sage
½ tablespoon of dried calendula
1 tablespoon of apricot oil
15 drops of rosemary essential oil

In a clean bowl mix the Epsom salts, dried herbs and apricot oil together, and then add the rosemary essential oil.

Pour into a 500ml clean, airtight container and use a table-spoonful each time you'd like a stimulating healing soak.

10. Rosemary and Sage Hair Rinse

Rosemary is a good astringent for oily hair and stimulating to hair follicles and growth.

3 sprigs of fresh rosemary
3 fresh sage leaves
15 drops of rosemary essential oil

Put the fresh herbs in a pot and pour on 3 cups of boiling water. Infuse for 15 minutes. Allow to cool until tepid and then add the essential oil.

After shampooing and rinsing, use this hair rinse, leaving it in for shining, beautiful healthy hair.

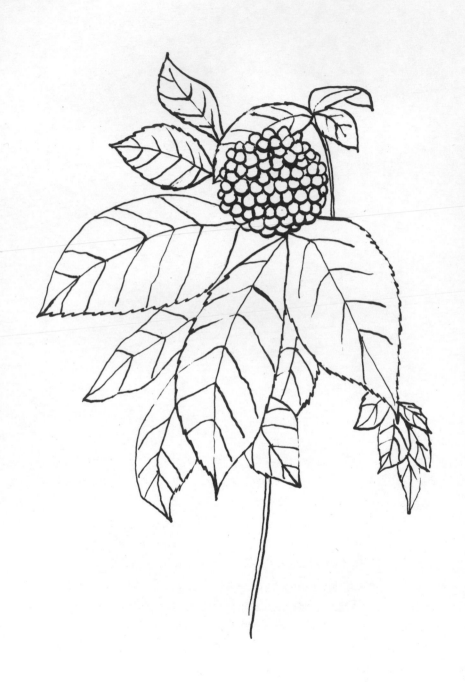

Siberian Ginseng

Eleutherococcus senticosus

Native to: East Asia, China, Russia

My favourite uses: for busy high flyers and multi-tasking parents, exhaustion or burn out, improving stamina, osteoarthritis, to help with the effects of jet lag, debilitating flu, to help mental focus

Siberian ginseng is also known as eleuthero, *ci wu jia* in Chinese and *ezoukogi* in Japanese. This adaptogen has almost the same properties as its cousin Panax ginseng and is from the Araliaceae ginseng family although eleuthero, rather confusingly, is not actually a ginseng.

This thorny creeping plant grows to around 3 metres in height and is very easy to grow as a hedge or border. The root is the main part used for its medicinal properties and these roots are extracted in late autumn when the active constituents are at their highest. The leaf is also medicinal and has a history of use as a poultice for inflammation.

The use of Siberian ginseng in traditional Chinese medicine can be traced back thousands of years. It is known as a primary adaptogen, generally used to prevent colds, flu, inflammation and respiratory infections, but also to increase energy levels and strengthen *qi*, the body's vital energy.

The use of Siberian ginseng in Russia only started during the Second World War, when extensive studies were made on the effects of this root on soldiers to boost their endurance and performance under the extremely stressful conditions of war. By the late 1960s it was known as the 'king of adaptogens' by the Russians, and was used regularly as a restorative herb all over the Soviet Union. The Soviet Olympic team found that it enhanced their stamina and performance and, like astragalus, made recovery time from any injury much shorter.

There are many products on the market so make sure that you buy from a reputable source, and that it contains eleuthero-sides – Siberian ginseng's main active ingredient.

How Siberian Ginseng Can Benefit You

Siberian ginseng contains steroidal glycosides known as eleuth-erosides, which are this herb's main component, as well as vitamin E and beta-carotene, which are strong antioxidants. Its roots are mineral-rich in calcium, phosphorus, potassium, mag-nesium, sodium, iron, zinc, copper and manganese, making this herb a nourishing supporter.

Siberian ginseng's main use is to help support the body in resisting stressors, whether they be emotional or physical, help-ing the body properly respond to stress in a more manageable way.

Although it has a long history in traditional Chinese medi-cine of supporting male virility, it is beneficial to both men and women, young and old; and although it can be stimulating it is still considered a gentle, balancing herb.

Mind

I would recommend Siberian ginseng to those who are working long hours, and not sleeping or replenishing their bodies enough, such as students who need help with stamina, learning and memory. City workers, night-shift workers and multi-tasking parents all need help focusing when burning the candle at both ends.

Those who are just exhausted by life's circumstances, physically and mentally stressed with a feeling of jangled nerves and forgetfulness, or who complain they 'can't think straight' might like to consider Siberian ginseng too. The herb will both support and protect.

If travelling on long haul flights regularly, Siberian ginseng will help protect against the negative effects of jet lag. It will help boost your short-term memory and concentration if you have to go straight from the airport into an important meeting.

Body

Siberian ginseng helps to improve your overall stamina, which makes it especially good for those multi-tasking with careers and family and the exhaustion this can bring, both mentally and physically.

Its nourishing tonic effects enhance the immune system, protecting the body from infection when you're feeling depleted. It also shortens the duration of illness if you do fall sick. Think of this herb if you're suffering from a debilitating chronic or stress-related illness such as chronic fatigue syndrome, Crohn's disease or hypertension.

This herb is being studied for its immune-modulating properties to see if it improves chemotherapy and radiation therapy and patients' recovery time afterwards. However, please speak to your oncologist before taking any herbal remedy or supplement, as it may interfere with your treatment.

Where there's chronic inflammation of the joints, Siberian ginseng has been found to be beneficial. A case study has shown improvement in the physical function, and relief from associated pain, with knee osteoarthritis.

Use Siberian ginseng to improve and support endurance and stamina in athletic performance. It also helps with recovery time in any injuries.

Beauty and Spirit

Siberian ginseng helps to prevent the feeling of being overwhelmed, anxious and exhausted. It will help with a general feeling of being grounded and connected when things feel completely out of control during stressful times, keeping the spirit balanced and calm, and encouraging a feeling of inner peace and strength.

Ten Ways with Siberian Ginseng

For best results, like all adaptogens, use over a period of time, preferably at the same time each day, for several weeks to a few months to get the optimum benefits. It takes about 3 weeks to have an effect and can be taken up to 3 months followed by a break of 3–4 weeks. It is best if children do not consume as it can be stimulating for sensitive people. If you are on medication consult your doctor before taking. Do not take with caffeine.

1. A Nerve Tonic Infusion

Combining tonic and nervine herbs to feed, strengthen and tone the nervous system. For this infusion I have combined chamomile flowers, which ease nervous tension, assisting with digestion; oat tops to help to feed the nervous system when exhausted, strengthening the system; nettle leaf strengthens, supports and nourishes the whole body; while of course the Siberian ginseng helps the body resist the negative effects of stress.

3 tablespoons of chamomile flowers (page 53)
2 tablespoons of oat tops (page 169)
2 tablespoons of nettle leaves (page 157)
1 tablespoon of Siberian ginseng (use the shredded root, not powdered)

In a clean, dry, airtight container mix together all the ingredients. When you are ready to infuse, add 3 teaspoons to a pot of hot water and allow to infuse for 15 minutes. Drink throughout the day, just keep adding boiling water.

2. A Refreshing, Simple Smoothie

1 banana
1 cup of yoghurt
1in piece of grated ginger
2 teaspoons of bee pollen (page 39)
1 dessertspoon of honey
1 teaspoon of ground Siberian ginseng

Blend the banana, yoghurt and ginger together. Then add the bee pollen, honey and Siberian ginseng and stir.

3. Compote, Chia and Siberian Ginseng Breakfast Pot

This breakfast pot is a truly delicious way to start your day. Chia seeds help to keep your energy levels balanced and the bowel regular, as they become gelatinous when soaked, helping with constipation.

4 tablespoons of chia seeds
400ml of almond milk
6 plums or apricots, stoned and quartered
1 dessertspoon of coconut sugar or agave syrup
1 dessertspoon of manuka honey
2 teaspoons of powdered Siberian ginseng

Combine the chia seeds and almond milk and leave to soak overnight, until the seeds are soaked and gelatinous.

Put the plums or apricots in a saucepan with enough water to cover the bottom. Simmer gently until the fruit is soft, then add the coconut sugar or agave syrup and stir. Remove from the heat and leave to cool.

The next morning, add some fruit compote to the chia seeds and stir in the manuka honey and Siberian ginseng.

4. Chai with a Difference

Add the following herbs to an airtight container to have a delicious supporting chai to hand.

6 tablespoons of green tea leaves (page 105)
4 slices of fresh ginger root, or 4 teaspoons of dried powdered
  ginger (page 81)
1 tablespoon of dried liquorice root (page 143)
1 tablespoon of dried Siberian ginseng

4 teaspoons of crushed cardamom
1 tablespoon of whole cloves
½ tablespoon of peppercorns

Gently warm 3 teaspoons of the herbs in a covered saucepan with 1 cup of filtered water for 15 minutes. Try not to boil the water. Strain the liquid into a teapot and add a little good quality honey, to taste.

Heat a cup of milk or milk substitute (I personally love soya or almond milk) and then pour a cup of half chai, half milk/almond milk, and sprinkle with a little nutmeg or cinnamon.

5. Brain Treats

The ingredients in these tasty energy balls help support cognitive function, improving memory, learning and mental fatigue. They also make a good pick-me-up for an afternoon slump.

1 tablespoon of good quality honey
1 tablespoon of almond butter
2 teaspoons of gotu kola powder
1 teaspoon of ginkgo powder
1 teaspoon of Siberian ginseng powder
1 cup of dried coconut flakes or desiccated coconut
½ cup of goji berries
Carob powder

Mix the honey and the almond butter together. Add the three powders and the coconut and berries, and then enough carob powder to make the mixture stiff enough to roll into balls.

Roll into balls in the palm of your hand and store in the fridge for up to three weeks. Eat one a day.

6. Elixir for Qi

Have a little tipple of this delicious elixir to keep the fire stoked and strong.

3 tablespoons of Siberian ginseng root
3 tablespoons of astragalus root
1 tablespoon of star anise
1 tablespoon of fresh ginger root or 3 teaspoons of dried ginger
1 tablespoon of liquorice root
Good quality brandy
Black cherry concentrate

Chop or break all the herbs down into small bits and place them in a wide-mouthed glass jar. Pour the brandy over to cover, and seal with a tight-fitting lid.

Let this sit for 6–8 weeks. Strain the liquid through a fine sieve or muslin and discard the herbs.

To every cup of elixir add ½ cup of black cherry concentrate and pour back into the jar. Give it a good shake.

Sip a small glass each day for a long life!

7. A Simple Decoction of Siberian Ginseng

Siberian ginseng has no bitter or pungent taste and therefore doesn't overpower the flavour of other herbs. So you could add ginger, lemon and cinnamon to this decoction if suffering from the flu or a cold, to add that extra anti-microbial, warming digestive effect.

Add 1 teaspoon of dried Siberian ginseng root to a few cups of filtered water in a saucepan. Simmer for 20 minutes, then allow to steep for an hour. Drink 3 times daily.

8. Supportive and Balancing Siberian Ginseng Tincture

Making a tincture of Siberian ginseng is the same as with the other root herbs in this book.

Finely cutting the root using a good knife, use enough to fill a quarter of your chosen clean, dry jar. Pour over the alcohol to the very top of the jar, covering the Siberian ginseng completely.

Leave this to macerate or soften over 4–6 weeks at room temperature, gently shaking the jar daily to allow the herb to mix with the alcohol.

Strain the herb from the liquid using muslin or a fine strainer, preserving the tincture in a new bottle. Label and date.

Use 30 drops, 3 times daily.

9. Rosemary and Siberian Ginseng Oil Rub

A great easy way to prepare a rub for sore joints and to get the circulation going.

1 cup of jojoba oil
1 tablespoon of vitamin E oil
20 drops of rosemary essential oil
30 drops of Siberian Ginseng Tincture (see above)

Mix together the oils and the tincture in a clean airtight container and label with the name and date.

Place a small amount in your palm and rub your hands together to warm the oil, then massage into aching joints.

Store at room temperature away from direct heat and sunlight for up to a year.

10. An Anti-ageing Soothing Face Mask

This homemade face mask makes perfect use of the healing and anti-ageing properties of Siberian ginseng. The wind- and sun-dried green clay from France can be sourced from Neal's Yard Remedies, or you can find suppliers online.

1 cup of green clay
3 teaspoons of powdered Siberian ginseng
½ cup of aloe vera juice
½ cup of mineral water

Blend everything together and paste on to a clean, dry face, avoiding the eyes. Leave until the clay dries. Rinse off with a face cloth and warm water.

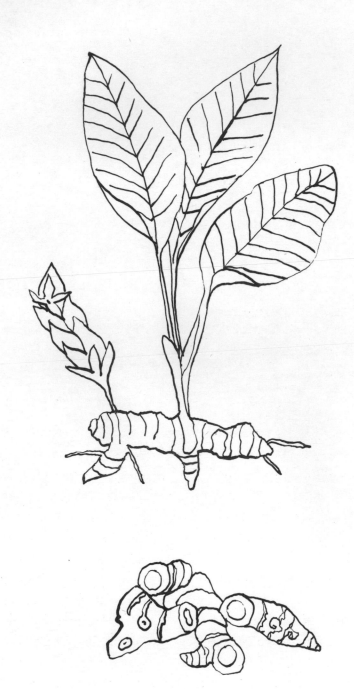

Turmeric

Curcuma longa

Native to: Southern Asia

My favourite uses: for inflammatory illnesses, poor digestion, chronic skin disorders, as an immune system enhancer

Turmeric has been used in Ayurvedic medicine for 4,000 years and has been known in Chinese medicine since the seventh century. This herb belongs to the Zingiberaceae family, otherwise known as the ginger family. It is thought to originate from Vietnam, China and Western India, but it is grown across the south of Asia including Indonesia and the Pacific Islands.

It's a perennial plant that grows over a metre tall. It needs a warm, tropical, humid environment with a good amount of rainfall in order to thrive. The roots and rhizomes (stems that grow underground), are the main parts used, which look very similar to ginger root and also are not dissimilar to caterpillar pupae.

Turmeric is most familiar as one of the ingredients in curry powder, and it is generally known for its culinary uses here in the West, adding that deep rich yellow colour and pungent bitter taste. It is ground with other spices as a base for curries.

Recently though its medicinal properties have come to light, and it is now being touted as the superherb for our everyday use. It is in fact a really accessible adaptogen that can be bought fresh in most health-food shops (and ground in every supermarket) and easily added to your daily routine.

In India and southern Asia turmeric has been used for thousands of years in cooking. It is eaten much like ginger, either cooked or eaten raw, although it is less fibrous than ginger. With its warming, stimulating properties which affect the whole digestive system, the fresh root can be chopped, or ground into a paste. Within Ayurvedic medicine it is used for warming the whole body system, improving not only digestion but arthritic joints and muscular pains.

Traditionally Hindus use turmeric every day to represent purity and prosperity. It is a valued herb in Hindu wedding ceremonies. A paste is prepared with turmeric, sandalwood and rosewater a few days before the wedding day and rubbed on the feet, knees, arms, hands and face of the bride and groom by a member of the family using mango leaves, to cleanse and protect the couple and ward off any evil from their future home. Known as the 'golden spice', turmeric is a symbol of the sun, fertility and purification, and is believed to relax the couple, lessening any pre-wedding nerves.

Its medicinal uses weren't considered in the West until the 1920s. And even then, generally Western herbalists have not thought to use this incredible herb until recently. Even the ancient Greeks, who had knowledge of this herb, preferred to use ginger root medicinally, and used turmeric mainly as a dye for clothes.

How Turmeric Can Benefit You

There seems to be no end to the healing potential of this golden spice.

In Okinawa, the islands of south Japan, the people enjoy the world's longest life expectancy. Men are usually expected to live to around 84, and women to almost 90. The inhabitants and many scientists attribute this to their diet, which is rich in soya, tofu, sea vegetables, sweet potato, brown rice, bitter melon – and turmeric, which they use every day in food and as infusions. Okinawans suffer half the dementia rates of Americans, and a fraction of the cardiovascular disease and prostate cancer.

Turmeric's main therapeutic constituents are the volatile oils known as curcuminoids, which give turmeric its beautiful, rich, fiery yellow pigment and its powerful biological properties. Curcumin is its primary curcuminoid and this constituent has been involved in recent studies to find out more about its therapeutic properties.

The only drawback is that curcumin only accounts for around 2–4 per cent of the constituents of turmeric so large amounts of the herb would need to be consumed in order to get enough effectual curcumin into the body. This is the reason people take curcumin extract in supplement form, but both curcumin and turmeric on their own are assimilated poorly by the body and eliminated quickly. Research therefore went into seeing how to make their medicinal benefits more available and it was found that piperine, an active ingredient in black pepper responsible for its pungent taste, was found to be what is known as a 'bio-enhancer'. When taken at the same time as taking whole turmeric and extracted curcumin supplements, piperine increases their bio-availability.

When looking at supplements, be sure that piperine is included in the ingredients, and when cooking with turmeric, be sure to add a good pinch of black pepper to the dish.

As a therapeutic dose you should take 2–8g of turmeric powder daily, added to food, or a fluid extract of 10ml daily. With curcumin, for a preventative everyday dose take 1,000mg daily, and up to 4,000mg daily as a therapeutic dose. As with most adaptogen herbs it usually takes up to eight weeks for the benefits to become apparent, so be patient in the first few weeks of taking turmeric.

Mind

In Asia there has been a study to prove something that Ayurvedic practitioners have known for centuries: that those people over the age of 60 who consumed curries containing turmeric on a regular, daily basis, with the herb's high antioxidant and anti-inflammatory properties, had a higher cognitive function than those who didn't eat turmeric daily.

In another clinical trial curcumin was found to be a safe and effective way of supporting patients with depression.

Turmeric has been shown to work directly with those who feel over-stressed and easily irritated, working with the stress response by helping to balance and support the adrenal glands. When the adrenals are constantly under stress this can trigger the body's autoimmune system and set off an inflammatory response.

Turmeric is believed to balance the emotions and is known to provide a feeling of inner strength. Taking turmeric daily is ideal to help clear negative energy and create a more positive outlook.

Body

Turmeric's potential is held in such high esteem that it is being used in clinical trials to test its efficacy against serious illnesses including Alzheimer's disease, diabetes, cancer and to inhibit HIV.

Curcuminoids have been found to be strong antioxidants, neutralising free radicals and protecting DNA against damage.

There have been many studies of curcumin and the effects this phytochemical has on cancer prevention and inhibiting the growth of cancer cells. Several studies report that curcumin can inhibit cancer cells from rapidly growing and induce apoptosis, a process of cell self-destruction, and, interestingly, around the globe people in the countries that use turmeric daily in their diet have lower levels of cancer than those in countries that don't routinely consume turmeric.

In animal tests, turmeric was found to protect against colon, stomach and skin cancers. Further human studies still need to be done, although in treating pancreatic cancer, curcumin along with chemotherapy has had positive early results (but with further studies to be done). A mixture of sandalwood and turmeric, however, was found to be of real benefit for those suffering from radiation dermatitis, a painful side effect from radiation treatment for head and neck cancers.

Important note

Always consult your oncologist before taking any herbs and supplements when undergoing chemotherapy and radiation therapy.

Recent studies have suggested that turmeric supplements and using turmeric in foods may interfere with the activity of some chemotherapy drugs used to treat breast cancer and should be avoided. Continuing studies are being done to see if turmeric is harmful during this treatment.

Turmeric has been used for centuries in Ayurvedic medicine and traditional Chinese medicine to treat arthritis and many other inflammatory diseases because of its amazing results. A recent study showed that its anti-inflammatory properties are so strong that it worked better than allopathic analgesic drugs in people with osteoarthritis, and without the usual side effects on the digestive system. Turmeric works by blocking the body's production of a protein that switches on a gene which tells blood vessels to form around inflammation, allowing it to grow. Essentially, turmeric stops inflammation in its tracks.

It also supports the muscles, strengthening connective tissue, and helps the body after prolonged illness or over-exertion when doing intensive physical training, helping to stimulate muscle renewal.

Use turmeric to protect, detoxify and regenerate the liver and to increase the flow of bile in the digestive system. This helps with the digestive process, and in detoxifying and rebalancing the whole body system. Make a decoction to relieve indigestion and soothe the stomach after a meal. Turmeric has also had positive results in treating more serious digestive problems such as ulcerated colitis and irritable bowel syndrome.

Turmeric can also help stimulate appetite after an illness or in illnesses related to appetite suppression, such as anorexia.

As an antibacterial it protects the body from salmonella and staphylococcus infection. It is especially good to take if the body is already compromised with a chronic illness, or when travelling to protect the digestive system from food poisoning.

Curcumin has been found to have an important role in the prevention and treatment of diabetes and the complications of this increasingly common disease, such as insulin resistance and hyperglycaemia.

Beauty and Spirit

With its high antioxidant levels, turmeric helps to protect the skin from premature ageing and environmental stressors, from pollution to too much sun exposure. Its microbial properties help to heal chronic irritated skin disorders such as psoriasis, and it has been used for centuries topically as an antibacterial in treating wounds, burns and skin infections.

Turmeric also protects and strengthens the eyes from age-degenerative disorders such as cataracts, working to prevent inflammation.

Ten Ways with Turmeric

Try to use organic turmeric if possible.

1. A Nourishing Cuppa

This is the perfect warming pick-me-up. In Okinawa, where they have the longest average lifespan of 81.2 years, they drink copious amounts of turmeric tea daily.

1 dessertspoon of grated turmeric
Grated skin and juice of half a lemon
1 dessertspoon of grated ginger (less if desired) (page 81)
3 peppercorns, slightly crushed
Organic honey, to taste

Mix all of the ingredients except the honey and place them in a pot of very hot water. Let them steep for 10–15 minutes.

Add a little more hot water and a dash of honey, to taste. Drink throughout the day.

2. A Super Smoothie

Try this smoothie for a get-up-and-go boost to your morning.

½ an avocado
1 cup of coconut water
1 cup of fresh spinach leaves
1 cup of berries of choice (I like raspberries or blueberries)
1 teaspoon of powered turmeric
½ teaspoon of powered ginger (page 81)
1 tablespoon of flax oil

Pulse all of the ingredients together in a blender and enjoy!

3. A Winter Soothing Warmer

Combine the following ingredients for a traditional cup of exotic golden milk.

1 teaspoon of powdered turmeric
1 teaspoon of almond oil
A splash of clear honey
200ml of almond milk, or milk of your choice

Mix the turmeric in a saucepan with the oil and the honey over a low heat, until the honey melts a little to form a paste, stirring with a whisk. Then slowly mix in a little bit of milk at a time, continuously stirring until all the milk has been added and the turmeric and honey have been mixed completely into the milk.

4. Scrambled Kale and Turmeric

Due to its mild, slightly bitter flavour, a dash of turmeric blends well with scrambled eggs to give your breakfast a golden twist. Add a pinch or more when stirring your eggs over the heat to add flavour and a medicinal zing.

1 dessertspoon of olive oil
A handful of kale
A dash of ground black pepper
A dash of salt
2 eggs
2 teaspoons of powdered turmeric

Put the oil in a saucepan and heat gently. Add the kale and sauté for 1 minute. Season with black pepper and salt.

Whisk the eggs with the turmeric, and add them to the pan and stir until just set.

Enjoy this healthy breakfast.

5. Curry Paste

To add a delicious traditional flavour to your curry.

3 tablespoons of coriander seeds
2 tablespoons of cumin seeds
1 tablespoon of mustard seeds
1 teaspoon of fennel seeds
1 teaspoon of black peppercorns
1 teaspoon of ground turmeric
1 teaspoon of ground cinnamon
1 teaspoon of paprika
1 or 2 dried chillies, depending on personal preference

1 teaspoon of salt
1 thumb-sized piece of root ginger, peeled and finely grated
  (page 81)
4 garlic cloves, crushed
1 tablespoon of tomato purée
4 tablespoons of white wine vinegar or cider vinegar
Vegetable or sunflower oil, to cover the paste for storing

Put the whole seeds and peppercorns into a dry frying pan over a medium heat. Cook for about 3 minutes, stirring often, until the mustard seeds start to pop and the seeds turn golden and aromatic. Tip into a bowl and allow to cool for a few minutes.

Put the turmeric, cinnamon, paprika and dried chillies into a pestle and mortar. Add the cooled toasted seeds and grind everything together into a fine powder. Add the salt.

Add the ginger, garlic, tomato purée and vinegar and mix well to make a paste.

Use immediately, or spoon the paste into a jar, cover with a layer of oil, seal with a lid and store in the fridge for up to a week.

6. A Flu Fighter

This is a great home remedy for when a nasty bug strikes, or when you want to boost your immunity when there's a virus outbreak.

¼ cup of cider vinegar
¼ cup of grated horseradish
1 onion, finely chopped
1 clove of garlic, crushed
3 teaspoons of powdered turmeric, or 5 medium rhizomes of
  grated fresh turmeric

1 pinch of cayenne pepper
1 pinch of ground black pepper
1 cup of organic honey (I like to use manuka)

Combine the vinegar, horseradish, onion, garlic, turmeric and a pinch of cayenne and black pepper together in a jar. Let this sit in a warm place for 3 weeks.

After 3 weeks, strain the mixture, add the honey and rebottle. Keep in the fridge for up to 4 weeks.

Take 1 tablespoon every 3 hours at the start of any cold or flu symptoms, and watch your immunity work wonders for you.

7. A Beneficial Tincture

A simple way of reaping the medicinal benefits of this fine adaptogen.

1 cup of peeled fresh turmeric, sliced or shredded
500ml of good brandy or vodka

Place the turmeric in a sterilised dry, glass jar, about two-thirds full. Pour over the alcohol, making sure the turmeric is completely covered. Place the lid on and store in a cool, dry, dark place for a few weeks. Shake the bottle gently every few days.

After a few weeks, strain the tincture into a bowl using a fine sieve or through muslin. Pour the tincture into amber bottles and don't forget to label and date them. This should keep for a few years. Use 30–40 drops three times a day.

You can also find a turmeric tincture from a reputable herbal company such as Neal's Yard Remedies.

8. A Sprain Soother

This paste helps to relieve inflammation and speeds up the healing process of sprains.

4 teaspoons of powdered turmeric
A good quality organic thick honey

Mix together and apply to the inflamed site twice a day, morning and night.

9. A Wound Cleanser

This is a wonderful remedy for when the immune system is compromised and run down and has manifested in boils and abscesses of the skin, or if you have a wound that just won't heal.

1 dessertspoon of turmeric powder
1 dessertspoon of ginger powder (page 81)

Combine the turmeric and ginger with enough cooled boiled water to make a paste.

Apply immediately to the affected area and cover with lint and then a cloth.

Put a hot water bottle on top for 5–15 minutes. Leave the paste on for half an hour in the morning, and in the evening, leaving on all night if possible.

10. Skin Clarifying Face Mask

Turmeric is high in antioxidants and helps to clarify and cleanse the skin, leaving it bright, smooth and even. Turmeric can stain your skin, but don't worry if there is any residue of yellow left on your face; wash it away with a little olive oil on a cotton pad. Wear something that's old and use a face cloth that you don't mind getting stained . . . just in case!

1 dessertspoon of good quality honey
1 dessertspoon of natural organic yoghurt
1 teaspoon of turmeric powder

Mix the ingredients together and apply a good layer to your whole face, avoiding the eyes.

Wash your hands and relax with cotton wool pads soaked in cold rosewater over your eyes for 20 minutes.

Rinse with a face cloth and warm water.

Suppliers and Stockists

Here are just a few of my favourite places to buy the adaptogens and ingredients mentioned in this book. Please do a little research to find a reputable supplier of herbs. I like to buy my herbs from companies that are organic, sustainable and fair trade, and a member of the Soil Association wherever possible.

Suppliers for herbs and other ingredients which I highly recommend and love are:

- Neal's Yard Remedies: www.nealsyardremedies.com
- The Organic Herb Trading Company: http://www. organicherbtrading.com
- Planet Organic: http://www.planetorganic.com
- Poyntzfield Herb Nursery: http://www.poyntzfieldherbs. co.uk
- For mushrooms: http://www.maesymush.co.uk
- For organic amla: http://aryanint.com

For bottles and harder to source supplies try:

- G. Balwin & Co: www.baldwins.co.uk
- Lakeland: http://www.lakeland.co.uk

A Note on Foraging

When foraging for rose hips, hawthorn, nettles, elderflowers and berries, try to choose a place away from busy polluted roads or by the side of farmed fields where pesticides may have been used.

Pick on a dry day in the morning, and make absolutely sure you have the right leaf and berry. A good reference book is Black's Nature Guide, *Medicinal Plants of Britain and Europe*. There are books about every region of the world to help you identify herbs native to your area.

References

General

Bartram's Encyclopedia of Herbal Medicine by Thomas Bartram
Culpeper's Complete Herbal by Nicholas Culpeper
Herbal Recipes for Vibrant Health by Rosemary Gladstar
Medicinal Mushrooms by Christopher Hobbs
The New Holistic Herbal by David Hoffmann
Hedgerow Medicine by Julie Bruton-Seal and Matthew Seal
Cooking Weeds by Vivien Weise
The Fragrant Pharmacy by Valerie Ann Worwood
Adaptogens in Medical Herbalism by Donald R. Yance

Amla

Akhtar MS, Ramzan A, Ali A, Ahmad M. Effect of Amla fruit (*Emblica officinalis* Gaertn.) on blood glucose and lipid profile of normal subjects and type 2 diabetic patients. *Int J Food Sci Nutr.* 2011 Sep; 62 (6): 609–16.

Damodara Reddy V, Padmavathi P, Gopi S, Paramahamsa M, Varadacharyulu N. Protective effect of *Emblica officinalis* against alcohol-induced hepatic injury by ameliorating oxidative stress in rats. *Pharm Biol.* 2011 Nov; 49 (11): 1128–36.

De A, De A, Papasian C, et al. *Emblica officinalis* extract induces autophagy and inhibits human ovarian cancer cell proliferation, angiogenesis, growth of mouse xenograft tumors. *PLoS One.* 2013 Aug 15; 8 (8): e72748.

Hiraganahalli BD, Chinampudur VC, Dethe S, et al. Hepatoprotective and antioxidant activity of standardized herbal extracts. *Pharmacogn Mag.* 2012 Apr; 8 (30): 116–23.

Jose JK, Kuttan G, Kuttan R. Antitumor activity of *Emblica officinalis. J Ethnopharmacol.* 2001; 75 (2–3): 65–9.

Piva R, Penolazzi L, Borgatti M, et al. Apoptosis of human primary osteoclasts treated with molecules targeting nuclear factor-kappa B. *Ann NY Acad Sci.* 2009 Aug; 1171: 448–56.

Yang CJ, Wang CS, Hung JY, et al. Pyrogallol induces G2-M arrest in human lung cancer cells and inhibits tumor growth in an animal model. *Lung Cancer.* 2009 Nov; 66 (2): 162–8.

Yokozawa T, Kim HY, Kim HJ, et al. Amla (*Emblica officinalis* Gaertn.) prevents dyslipidaemia and oxidative stress in the ageing process. *Br J Nutr.* 2007; 97 (6): 1187–95.

Bee Pollen

Al-Waili N, Al-Ghamdi A, Ansari MJ, et al. Synergistic effects of honey and propolis toward drug multi-resistant *Staphylococcus aureus, Escherichia coli* and *Candida albicans* isolates in single and polymicrobial cultures. *Int J Med Sci.* 2012; 9 (9): 793–800.

Kamiya T, Nishihara H, Hara H, et al. Ethanol extract of Brazilian red propolis induces apoptosis in human breast cancer MCF-7 cells through endoplasmic reticulum stress. *J Agric Food Chem.* 2012 Nov 7; 60 (44): 11065–70.

Kumazaki M, Shinohara H, Taniguchi K, et al. Propolis cinnamic acid derivatives induce apoptosis through both extrinsic and intrinsic apoptosis signaling pathways and modulate of miRNA expression. *Phytomedicine.* 2014 Jul–Aug; 21 (8–9): 1070–77.

Pascoal A, Rodrigues S, Teixeira A, Feás X, Estevinho LM. Biological activities of commercial bee pollens: antimicrobial, antimuta-genic, antioxidant and anti-inflammatory. *Food Chem Toxicol.* 2014 Jan; 63: 233–9.

Sun LP, Chen AL, Hung HC, et al. Chrysin: a histone deacetylase 8 inhibitor with anticancer activity and a suitable candidate for the standardization of Chinese propolis. *J Agric Food Chem*. 2012 Nov 28; 60 (47): 11748–58.

Szliszka E, Zydowicz G, Mizgala E, et al. Artepillin C (3,5-diprenyl-4-hydroxycinnamic acid) sensitizes LNCaP prostate cancer cells to TRAIL-induced apoptosis. *Int J Oncol*. 2012 Sep; 41 (3): 818–28.

Wang K, Zhang J, Ping S, et al. Anti-inflammatory effects of ethanol extracts of Chinese propolis and buds from poplar (*Populus* x *canadensis*). *J Ethnopharmacol*. 2014 Aug 8; 155 (1): 300–311.

Wu J, Omene C, Karkoszka J, et al. Caffeic acid phenethyl ester (CAPE), derived from a honeybee product propolis, exhibits a diversity of anti-tumor effects in pre-clinical models of human breast cancer. *Cancer Lett*. 2011 Sep 1; 308 (1): 43–53.

Chamomile

Al-Hashem FH. Gastroprotective effects of aqueous extract of *Chamomilla recutita* against ethanol-induced gastric ulcers. *Saudi Med J*. 2010 Nov; 31 (11): 1211–16.

Arango D, Morohashi K, Yilmaz A, et al. Molecular basis for the action of a dietary flavonoid revealed by the comprehensive identification of apigenin human targets. *Proc Natl Acad Sci USA*. 2013 Jun 11; 110 (24): E2153–62.

Keefe JR, Mao JJ, Soeller I, Li QS, Amsterdam JD. Short-term open-label chamomile (*Matricaria chamomilla* L.) therapy of moderate to severe generalized anxiety disorder. *Phytomedicine*. 2016 Dec 15; 23 (14): 1699–1705.

Mao JJ, Xie SX, Keefe JR, Soeller I, Li QS, Amsterdam JD. Long-term chamomile (*Matricaria chamomilla* L.) treatment for generalized anxiety disorder: A randomized clinical trial. *Phytomedicine*. 2016 Dec 15; 23 (14): 1735–42.

Patel D, Shukla S, Gupta S. Apigenin and cancer chemoprevention: progress, potential and promise (review). *Int J Oncol*. 2007 Jan; 30 (1): 233–45.

Rafraf M, Zemestani M, Asghari-Jafarabadi M. Effectiveness of chamomile tea on glycemic control and serum lipid profile in patients with type 2 diabetes. *J Endocrinol Invest.* 2014 Sep 7.

Srivastava JK, Gupta S. Antiproliferative and apoptotic effects of chamomile extract in various human cancer cells. *J Agric Food Chem.* 2007 Nov 14; 55 (23): 9470–78.

Srivastava JK, Pandey M, Gupta S. Chamomile, a novel and selective COX-2 inhibitor with anti-inflammatory activity. *Life Sci.* 2009 Nov 4; 85 (19–20): 663–9.

Elderberry

Krawitz C, Mraheil MA, Stein M, et al. Inhibitory activity of a standardized elderberry liquid extract against clinically-relevant human respiratory bacterial pathogens and influenza A and B viruses. *BMC Complement Altern Med.* 2011; 11: 16.

Scopel M, Mentz LA, Henriques AT. Comparative analysis of *Sambucus nigra* and *Sambucus australis* flowers: development and validation of an HPLC method for raw material quantification and preliminary stability study. *Planta Med.* 2010 Jul; 76 (10): 1026–31.

Thole JM, Kraft TF, Sueiro LA, et al. A comparative evaluation of the anticancer properties of European and American elderberry fruits. *J Med Food.* 2006 Winter; 9 (4): 498–504.

Zakay-Rones Z, Thom E, Wollan T, et al. Randomized study of the efficacy and safety of oral elderberry extract in the treatment of influenza A and B virus infections. *J Int Med Res.* 2004 Mar–Apr; 32 (2): 132–40.

Zakay-Rones, Mumcuoglu, et al. Inhibition of several strains of influenza virus in vitro and reduction of symptoms by an elderberry extract (Sambucus nigra L.) during an outbreak of influenza B Panama. *J Altern Complement Med.* 1995 Winter; 1(4): 361–9.

Ginger

Daily JW, Zhang X, Kim da S, Park S. Efficacy of ginger for alleviating the symptoms of primary dysmenorrhea: a systematic review and meta-analysis of randomized clinical trials. *Pain Med.* 2015 Dec; 16 (12): 2243–55.

Grøntved A, Brask T, Kambskard J, Hentzer E. Ginger root against seasickness. A controlled trial on the open sea. *Acta Otolaryngol.* 1988 Jan–Feb; 105 (1–2): 45–9.

Levine ME, Gillis MG, Koch SY, et al. Protein and ginger for the treatment of chemotherapy-induced delayed nausea. *J Altern Complement Med.* 2008 Jun; 14 (5): 545–51.

Oboh G, Ademiluyi AO, Akinyemi AJ. Inhibition of acetylcholinesterase activities and some pro-oxidant induced lipid peroxidation in rat brain by two varieties of ginger (*Zingiber officinale*). *Exp Toxicol Pathol.* 2012 May; 64 (4): 315–19.

Pillai AK, Sharma KK, Gupta YK, et al. Anti-emetic effect of ginger powder versus placebo as an add-on therapy in children and young adults receiving high emetogenic chemotherapy. *Pediatr Blood Cancer.* 2011 Feb; 56 (2): 234–8.

Podlogar JA, Verspohl EJ. Antiinflammatory effects of ginger and some of its components in human bronchial epithelial (BEAS-2B) cells. *Phytother Res.* 2012 Mar; 26 (3): 333–6.

Saenghong N, Wattanathorn J, Muchimapura S, Tongun T, Piyavhatkul N, Banchonglikitkul C, Kajsongkram T. *Zingiber officinale* improves cognitive function of the middle-aged healthy women. *Evid Based Complement Alternat Med.* 2011 Dec 22; doi 10.1155/2012/383062.

Zeng GF, Zhang ZY, Lu L, et al. Protective effects of ginger root extract on Alzheimer disease-induced behavioral dysfunction in rats. *Rejuvenation Res.* 2013 Apr; 16 (2): 124–33.

Gotu Kola

Jana U, Sur TK, Maity LN, Debnath PK, Bhattacharyya D. A clinical study on the management of generalized anxiety disorder with *Centella asiatica*. *Nepal Med Coll J.* 2010 Mar; 12 (1): 8–11.

Paocharoen V. The efficacy and side effects of oral *Centella asiatica* extract for wound healing promotion in diabetic wound patients. *J Med Assoc Thai.* 2010 Dec; 93 Suppl 7: S166–70.

Soumyanath A, Zhong YP, Henson E, et al. *Centella asiatica* extract improves behavioral deficits in a mouse model of Alzheimer's disease: investigation of a possible mechanism of action. *Int J Alzheimers Dis.* 2012; e381974.

Tang XL, Yang XY, Jung HJ, et al. Asiatic acid induces colon cancer cell growth inhibition and apoptosis through mitochondrial death cascade. *Biol Pharm Bull.* 2009 Aug; 32 (8): 1399–405.

Wattanathorn J, Mator L, Muchimapura S, et al. Positive modulation of cognition and mood in the healthy elderly volunteer following the administration of *Centella asiatica. J Ethnopharmacol.* 2008 Mar 5; 116 (2): 325–32.

Green Tea

Hsu SD, et al. Chemoprevention of oral cancer by green tea. *Gen Dent.* 2002; 50: 140–46.

Kuriyama S, Shimazu T, Ohmori K, Kikuchi N, Nakaya N, Nishino Y, Tsubono Y, Tsuji I. Green tea consumption and mortality due to cardiovascular disease, cancer, and all causes in Japan: the Ohsaki study. *JAMA* 2006; 296: 1255–65.

Nechuta S, Shu XO, Li HL, et al. Prospective cohort study of tea consumption and risk of digestive system cancers: results from the Shanghai Women's Health Study. *Am J Clin Nutr.* 2012 Nov; 96 (5): 1056–63.

Pisters KM, et al. Phase I trial of oral green tea extract in adult patients with solid tumors. *J Clin Oncol.* 2001; 19: 1830–38.

Proniuk S, et al. Preformulation study of epigallocatechin gallate, a promising antioxidant for topical skin cancer prevention. *J Pharm Sci.* 2002; 91: 111–16.

Rosetti F, Ferrari N, De Flora S. Angioprevention: angiogenesis is a common and key target for cancer chemopreventive agents. *FASEB J.* 2002; 16: 2–14.

Sartippour MR, et al. Green tea inhibits vascular endothelial growth factor (VEGF) induction in human breast cancer cells. *J Nutr.* 2002; 132: 2307–11.

Schmidt A, Hammann F, Wölnerhanssen B, et al. Green tea extract enhances parieto-frontal connectivity during working memory processing. *Psychopharmacology (Berl.)* 2014 Oct; 231 (19): 3879–88.

Sun CL, et al. Urinary tea polyphenols in relation to gastric and esophageal cancers: a prospective study of men in Shanghai, China. *Carcinogenesis* 2002; 23: 1497–503.

Liquorice

Al-Turki AI, El-Ziney MG, Abdel-Salam AM. Chemical and anti-bacterial characterization of aqueous extracts of oregano, marjoram, sage and licorice and their application in milk and labneh. *J Food Agric Environ.* 2008; 6: 39–44.

Awandkar SP, Mendhe MS, Badukale DM, Kulkarni MB. Antimicrobial action of cold aqueous and cold ethanolic extracts of *Glycyrrhiza glabra* against bovine mammary pathogens. *Anim Sci Rep.* 2012; 6: 88–91.

Bodet C, La VD, Gafner S, Bergeron C, Grenier D. A licorice extract reduces lipopolysaccharide-induced proinflammatory cytokine secretion by macrophages and whole blood. *J Periodontol.* 2008; 79: 1752–61.

Fujisawa K, Tandon BN. Therapeutic approach to the chronic active liver disease: Summary of a satellite symposium. In: Nishioka K, Suzuki H, Mishiro S, Oda T eds. *Viral Hepatitis and Liver Disease.* (Tokyo: Springer, 1994), 662–5.

Long DR, Mead J, Hendricks JM, Hardy ME, Voyich JM. 18β-Glycyrrhetinic acid inhibits methicillin-resistant *Staphylococcus aureus* survival and attenuates virulence gene expression. *Antimicrob Agents Chemother.* 2013; 57: 241–7.

Park IK, Kim J, Lee YS, Shin SC. *In vivo* fungicidal activity of medicinal plant extracts against six phytopathogenic fungi. *Int J Pest Manag.* 2008; 54: 63–8.

Nettle

Jacquet A, Girodet PO, Pariente A, et al. Phytalgic, a food supplement, vs placebo in patients with osteoarthritis of the knee or hip: a randomised double-blind placebo-controlled clinical trial. *Arthritis Res Ther.* 2009; 11 (6): R192.

Kianbakht S, Khalighi-Sigaroodi F, Dabaghian FH. Improved glycemic control in patients with advanced type 2 diabetes mellitus taking *Urtica dioica* leaf extract: a randomized double-blind placebo-controlled clinical trial. *Clin Lab.* 2013; 59 (9–10): 1071–6.

Konrad L, Muller HH, Lenz C, et al. Antiproliferative effect on human prostate cancer cells by a stinging nettle root (*Urtica dioica*) extract. *Planta Med.* 2000 Feb; 66 (1): 44–7. doi 10.1055/s-2000-11117.

Ozkol H, Musa D, Tuluce Y, et al. Ameliorative influence of *Urtica dioica* L against cisplatin-induced toxicity in mice bearing Ehrlich ascites carcinoma. *Drug Chem Toxicol.* 2012 Jul; 35 (3): 251–7. doi 10.3109/01480545.2011.598531.

Randall C, Randall H, Dobbs F, et al. Randomized controlled trial of nettle sting for treatment of base-of-thumb pain. *J R Soc Med.* 2000 Jun; 93 (6): 305–9.

Roschek B Jr., Fink RC, McMichael M, et al. Nettle extract (*Urtica dioica*) affects key receptors and enzymes associated with allergic rhinitis. *Phytother Res.* 2009 Jul; 23 (7): 920–26. doi 10.1002/ptr.2763.

Sayhan MB, Kanter M, Oguz S, et al. Protective effect of *Urtica dioica* L. on renal ischemia/reperfusion injury in rat. *J Mol Histol.* 2012 Dec; 43 (6): 691–8. doi 10.1007/s10735-012-9436-9.

Reishi

Chan WK, Cheung CC, Law HK, et al. *Ganoderma lucidum* polysaccharides can induce human monocytic leukemia cells into dendritic cells with immuno-stimulatory function. *J Hematol Oncol.* 2008; 1 (1): 9.

Chen NH, Liu JW, Zhong JJ. Ganoderic acid Me inhibits tumor invasion through down-regulating matrix metalloproteinases 2/9 gene expression. *J Pharmacol Sci.* 2008 Oct; 108 (2): 212–16.

Li YB, Wang R, Wu HL, et al. Serum amyloid A mediates the inhibitory effect of *Ganoderma lucidum* polysaccharides on tumor cell adhesion to endothelial cells. *Oncol Rep.* 2008 Sep;20 (3): 549–56.

Mao T, van de Water J, Keen CL, et al. Two mushrooms, *Grifola frondosa* and *Ganoderma lucidum*, can stimulate cytokine gene expression and proliferation in human T lymphocytes. *Int J Immunother.* 1999; 15 (1): 13–22.

Noguchi M, Kakuma T, Tomiyasu K, et al. Effect of an extract of *Ganoderma lucidum* in men with lower urinary tract symptoms: a double-blind, placebo-controlled randomized and dose-ranging study. *Asian J Androl.* 2008 Jul; 10 (4): 651–8.

Weng CJ, Yen GC. The in vitro and in vivo experimental evidences disclose the chemopreventive effects of *Ganoderma lucidum* on cancer invasion and metastasis. *Clin Exp Metastasis.* 2010 May; 27 (5): 361–9.

Rhodiola

de Bock K, Eijnde BO, Ramaekers M, et al. Acute *Rhodiola rosea* intake can improve endurance exercise performance. *Int J Sport Nutr Exerc Metab.* 2004 Jun; 14 (3): 298–307.

Darbinyan V, Kteyan A, Panossian A, et al. *Rhodiola rosea* in stress induced fatigue – a double blind cross-over study of a standardized extract SHR-5 with a repeated low-dose regimen on the mental performance of healthy physicians during night duty. *Phytomedicine.* 2000 Oct; 7 (5): 365–71.

van Diermen D, Marston A, Bravo J, et al. *Monoamine oxidase inhibition by Rhodiola rosea* L. roots. *J Ethnopharmacol.* 2009 Mar 18; 122 (2): 397–401.

Edwards D, Heufelder A, Zimmermann A. Therapeutic effects and safety of *Rhodiola rosea* extract WS® 1375 in subjects with life-stress symptoms – results of an open-label study. *Phytother Res.* 2012 Aug; 26 (8): 1220–25.

Ishaque S, Shamseer L, Bukutu C, Vohra S. *Rhodiola rosea* for physical and mental fatigue: a systematic review. *BMC Complement Altern Med.* 2012 May 29; 12: 70.

Shevtsov VA, Zholus BI, Shervarly VI, et al. A randomized trial of two different doses of a SHR-5 *Rhodiola rosea* extract versus placebo and control of capacity for mental work. *Phytomedicine.* 2003 Mar; 10 (2–3): 95–105.

Rose Hips

Christensen R, Sørensen LB, Bartels EM, Astrup A, Bliddal H. Rose-hip in osteoarthritis (OA): a meta-analysis. *Ann Rheum Dis.* 2007; 66 (Suppl II): 495.

Turmeric

Bundy R, Walker AF, Middleton RW, et al. Turmeric extract may improve irritable bowel syndrome symptomatology in otherwise healthy adults: a pilot study. *J Altern Complement Med.* 2004 Dec; 10 (6): 1015–18.

Dhillon N, Aggarwal BB, Newman RA, et al. Phase II trial of curcumin in patients with advanced pancreatic cancer. *Clin Cancer Res.* 2008 Jul 15;14 (14): 4491–9.

Hanai H, Iida T, Takeuchi K, et al. Curcumin maintenance therapy for ulcerative colitis: randomized, multicenter, double-blind, placebo-controlled trial. *Clinical Gastroenterol Hepatol.* 2006 Dec; 4 (12): 1502–6.

Kuptniratsaikul V, Dajpratham P, Taechaarpornkul W, et al. Efficacy and safety of *Curcuma domestica* extracts compared with ibuprofen in patients with knee osteoarthritis: a multicenter study. *Clin Interv Aging.* 2014 Mar 20; 9: 451–8.

Ng TP, Chiam PC, Lee T, et al. Curry consumption and cognitive function in the elderly. *Am J Epidemiol.* 2006 Nov 1; 164 (9): 898–906.

Palatty PL, Azmidah A, Rao S, et al. Topical application of a sandalwood oil and turmeric based cream prevents radiodermatitis in head and neck cancer patients undergoing external beam radiotherapy: a pilot study. *Br J Radiol.* 2014 Jun; 87 (1038): 20130490.

Sanmukhani J, Satodia V, Trivedi J, et al. Efficacy and safety of curcumin in major depressive disorder: a randomized controlled trial. *Phytother Res.* 2014 Apr; 28 (4): 579–85.

Shapiro K, Gong WC. Natural products used for diabetes. *J Am Pharm Ass*. 2002; 42 (2): 217–26.

Somasundaram S, Edmund NA, Moore DT, et al. Dietary curcumin inhibits chemotherapy-induced apoptosis in models of human breast cancer. *Cancer Res*. 2002 Jul 1; 62 (13): 3868–75.

Wu SH, Hang LW, Yang JS, et al. Curcumin induces apoptosis in human non-small cell lung cancer NCI-H460 cells through ER stress and caspase cascade- and mitochondria-dependent pathways. *Anticancer Res*. 2010 Jun; 30 (6): 2125–33.

Acknowledgements

I'd like to thank Angela and Peter Bradbury, my first teachers, who encouraged and inspired me along the way. Also Christopher and Non Hedley who taught me how to connect with herbs and introduced me to their many different personalities.

Thanks to my beautiful mum Agnes Beryl for sharing those special times in the chaos of her work and child-rearing. To my husband Charlie for all his support, patience and love.

And to my whole family, the greatest teachers of all, who each in their own individual way inspire me every day.

Thank you also to Jillian Young, my editor, for taking me on this special journey of *Superherbs*.

Index

About the Author

Rachel Landon is a Naturopath Iridologist and Herbalist. She is a member of the Association of Master Herbalists, with a private practice in North West London, where she specialises in family health, encouraging and inspiring clients to be active participants in their own health and well-being. She is currently creating a line of organic and wildcrafted botanical formulas that holistically support vitality and wellness.